D0804416

# Irisn Babies' Names

HarperCollins*Publishers*,
Westerhill Road, Bishopbriggs, Glasgow G64 2QT
www.collins.co.uk

First published 1996
This edition published 2004

Reprint 10 9 8 7 6 5 4 3

© Julia Cresswell, 2004

ISBN  0-00-7176171

Collins Gem® is a registered trademark of
HarperCollins*Publishers* Limited

Printed in Italy by Amadeus S.p.A.

# Contents

# Style of the entries

commonest form
of the name

Irish form of the name
(where applicable)

gender

**Alva** *Almha* f.
The meaning of this name is not known. Alva
was one of the Tuatha Dé Danann (see **Dana**)
who gave her name, in its old form *Almu*,
to the hill and its fortress at Almu in
Leinster.

bold italic text shows
another form of the
name

bold text cross-refers
to another entry

# Introduction

Irish names are spreading across the world. As well as being more common in Ireland itself, they have featured in the most-popular names lists in most English-speaking countries for decades, and recently even France was conquered, when Kevin became the most popular baby boy's name there.

The reason for this spread is not hard to find. Massive emigration, especially during the nineteenth-century famines, left many people of Irish descent in Britain, the USA, Canada and Australia. This Irish diaspora often had to give up the Irish language in favour of English, but they took their names with them, gave them to their children and spread them in the new countries. Indeed some, such as Brian, are now so well-established that they are no longer considered Irish. Others have developed strong associations with their new countries, so that Oscar is sometimes thought of as Scandinavian, Barry and Sheila are associated with Australia, and for most people Darren is American.

## Defining an Irish name

What then is an Irish name? In this book a very broad view is taken, with special attention paid to what has happened to names after they left Ireland.

**Gaelic names** The main category of names comes from the native Irish language (Gaelic), and purists might argue these are the only truly Irish names. Many come in at least two forms: the true native Irish form, and the anglicized form, reflecting the English rather than Irish pronunciation and spelling system. As the anglicized forms are generally the ones most widely used, I have usually listed the names under these forms, although every possible spelling has been cross-referenced. Thus, the name Kevin is discussed under this anglicized form, rather than under its true Irish spelling, *Caoimhín*.

**Translations** In the past, efforts were made to end Irish resistance to British rule by strangling the Irish language, and the use of Irish names was officially discouraged. As a result some Irish names have acquired equivalents taken from the common pool of European names. Where these are unusual outside Ireland, they too can be thought of as a class of Irish names. Thus the saint's name Thaddeus was used as a substitute for the Irish Tadhg, Ulysses used for Ulick and Unity for Una. These names are still more common in Ireland than elsewhere. I have used the term 'translation' for this class of name.

**Irish forms of non-Irish names** Another group is those names from other languages that have been given Irish forms. These are often saints' names which give us some of the best-known Irish names, such as Maire from Mary and Kathleen or Caitlin from Catherine. There is also a minor group of saints' names, such as Philomena, which have not been given Irish form but are far more popular in Catholic Ireland than the rest of the English-speaking world, and so can be thought of as predominantly Irish in usage. There are also Irish forms of a few non-Irish names that are not specifically religious in origin, such as Liam from William and Redmond, the Irish form of Raymond. A number of these were borrowed from the Vikings who raided then settled in Ireland from the eighth century.

*Irish surnames and words* Finally, many names originate Ireland but are much more likely to be found in other English-speaking countries. These are mostly Irish surnames such as Kelly and Ryan, often themselves based on earlier Irish first names and then been adopted as first names directly from the surname. A smaller number are from Irish words which are not used as names in Ireland, but which have been used particularly in the USA and Australia – typical of these are Kerry and Colleen.

*Terminology used in this book*
By Ireland I mean the whole island. Britain is,

of course, England, Scotland and Wales. Irish is used for the language otherwise called Gaelic. This is a Celtic language, Celtic referring both to the group of related languages derived from a common root and including Scots Gaelic, Welsh, Breton and the Gaulish language spoken in France before the Roman conquest; and to the culture of the Celtic peoples who once spread from Galicia (in modern Turkey) in the east to Ireland in the west. I have also described some names as coming from Germanic roots. This refers to the group of languages formerly spoken by the northern peoples and which developed into, among other languages, modern German and English. It lay behind the languages of the Vikings and the Franks, who conquered France after the fall of the Roman Empire.

### Meanings of names

Where possible I have given the meanings of names. This involves looking at their earliest forms, for language changes over the centuries and meanings cannot always be deduced from names' modern forms. For example, Donovan is *Donnabhán* in Irish, which very much looks as if it is made up of the elements *donn*, 'brown', and *bhán* 'white'. But in fact the old form of the name is *Donndubán*, with the second part of the name coming from *dub* 'black, dark', so the name means 'dark brown' rather than 'light brown'. Many names have traditional meanings that the language experts now say are not correct. However, the 'meaning' of a name is really a loose idea, and what you think a name really 'means' is just as important as what scholars consider it to mean. People should feel free to choose a name for its personal associations and meanings for them and their friends.

## Spelling variations

Historical circumstance has left many Irish names with several spellings. The relatively small numbers who could both speak and write Irish in the nineteenth century coupled with regional variations in pronunciation meant that those wishing to use the old Irish names again had to work out spellings for themselves. The resulting variations were further compounded by spelling reforms introduced in the mid-twentieth century. In addition, attempts to anglicize the names, often using phonetic spellings based on the word sound, have also meant that the resulting spellings can be very different from the original names. Finally, some saints' names have been filtered through Latin, and have taken on yet other forms. I have tried to include as many of these variations as possible, emphasising the forms that are used today but including those which might be found in history books or stories of the saints.

The nicest part of an introduction to write is the thank yous. I should like to thank my commissioning editor James Carney, whose idea the book was, and his production team; Barry Riordan, teacher of Irish, who looked at portions of the text and corrected my Irish – any remaining mistakes are entirely mine – and who provided some of the best stories, and John Brophy and Louise Ni Chriodain who provided the pronunciations for the names. I should also like to thank Fred McDonald for the sustaining phone calls, my husband Philip who read portions of the text and told me if it made sense, and my son Alexander for his patience in accepting that I was not available to do much better things like being with him.

*Julia Cresswell*
*2004*

# *a*

**Adamair** *see* **Aodh**

**Adamnan** *ádhamhnán m.*

The meaning of this name is not entirely clear: it is generally interpreted as a pet form of **Adam** (*Ádhamh*), but scholars now think it comes from an old Irish word meaning 'fear' and means something like 'frightened one', or as one commentator has suggested, 'little horror'. Its most famous bearer was St Adamnan or *Adomnan*, abbot of Iona (627–704). He was a great church and social reformer who introduced the Law of Adomnan (*Cain Adomnain*), accepted across Ireland in times of war, which ruled that all women, children and those in holy orders should be regarded as non-combatants. He was also a noted author, being particularly famous for his life of St **Columba** (see **Colm**), founder of the monastery on Iona, and left us our first mention

11

of the Loch Ness Monster. The name was frequently anglicized as *Eunan*, which follows the Irish pronunciation, or *Onan*, and is also found as *Awnan*, *Odanodan*, *Ounan*, and even as *Junan* or *Junanan*.

### Aed *see* Aodh

### Aedan *see* Aidan

### Aeneas *see* Aengus, Eneas

### Aengus *Aonghus* m.

Aengus can be interpreted as meaning 'one choice' or 'true vigour'. It is the Irish form of the name better known in its Scottish form *Angus* (a form also found in Ireland), although Yeats' delightful poem *The Song of Wandering Aengus* has introduced the Irish version to a world-wide audience. *Óengus*, *Aonghas* and *Áengus* are alternative Irish spellings, and the name was sometimes anglicized phonetically as *Eenis*, and *Aeneas* or *Eneas*, the name of the great Trojan hero, used as a translation (see that entry for more details). The Irish pronunciation gave rise to forms such as *Neese*, *Neece* or *Niece*, and *Enos* is also found. There is a rare female form, *Angustina*. The original Aengus was one of the great gods of the Irish, the son of the *Dagda* (see **Dáire**) and the goddess of the River Boyne. He was a god of youth and of love, and is shown in stories helping the two most famous pairs of lovers in Irish romance, **Etain** and Midhir, and **Dermot** and **Grania**. He himself had many loves, one of the most famous being found in the old story called *The Dream of Aengus*, where he became sick with love for a girl he saw repeatedly in his dreams, and suffered many adventures to win her. Another Aengus became the first Christian king of Cashel in 490, some thirty years after the death of St **Patrick**.

### Ághaistín, Aibhistín *see* Augusteen

### Aghna, Agnes *see* Ina

### Aibhilín *see* Aileen, Eileen, Evelyn

### Aibhne *see* Eveny

### Aidan *Aodán, Aodhan* m.

This name means 'little fire' and is a pet form of **Aodh**. Its most famous bearer, St Aidan (d. 651), left the great monastery on Iona where he was a monk to go to Northumbria at the request of King Oswald, who had himself been an exile on Iona.

Oswald gave him the island of Lindisfarne where Aidan founded the famous monastery to use as a base to convert the pagan Saxons to Christianity. We know little of Aidan's life before this time other than that he was Irish, but his ministry in the north of England is well documented by the Venerable Bede (673–735), who praised him for his love of prayer and study, and for his peacefulness and humility. Because of his connections with northern England the name has been used there, and currently seems to be becoming more popular in Britain as a whole. The name was popular among the Irish in the past – there are at least twenty-one saints called Aidan, of whom Aidan of Lindisfarne is the best known – and is popular in Ireland again today. It is often spelt **Aedan**, and is also found as **Aiden** and **Edan**. Aidan and **Aida** have been used as girls' names, but **Edana** is a more usual feminine form. (See also **Ena** and **Enat**.)

### Aignéis *see* Ina

### Ailbe, Ailbhe *see* Alby

### Aileen *Aibhílín* f
This is a currently popular form of **Eileen** (under which more information is given) or *Eibhlín*, an

Irish form of **Evelyn** or *Aveline*, a name brought
to Ireland by the Normans. It is also found in the
spelling *Ailine*, and particularly in the USA, *Ailene*
and *Ailleen*. (See also **Aline**.)

## Ailis *Ailís, Ailíse f.*

These are the Irish forms of *Alice* and *Alicia*, names
brought by the Normans and which come from a
word meaning 'noble'. Ailis can also be found in the
phonetic spelling *Ailish*, although many users
probably regard Ailish as an alternative spelling of
the more common *Eilish* (see **Eilis**).

## Ailleen *see* Aileen

## Aindrias, Aindriú *m.*

These are the Irish forms of the name of the
apostle Andrew. The original name was Greek and
means 'manly'. Andrew is also found as *Aindréas*.

## Áine *f.*

Áine, which means 'brightness, splendour', seems
originally to have been a title used by both gods
and goddesses, but is now only used as a female
name. There is a well-known Áine who figures in
Irish folklore, and the name crops up throughout
Ireland, but the best-known stories are associated

with the goddess Áine's fairy hill of Knockainey (Cnoc Áine) in Co. Limerick, and with the kings of Munster, who claimed her as an ancestress. This Áine was later adopted by the conquering Norman Fitzgerald family (see further under **Geraldine**), who also claimed her as an ancestress, and the name Áine Fitzgerald is still to be found today. In other stories she is human rather than from the other-world, and is described as 'the best-hearted woman who ever lived'. The name can also be used in combination, as in the case of the Irish traditional singer Maire Áine ni Dhonnchada. It was translated Ann(e) or Anna in the past, and many Irish people still regard Áine as the Irish form of these names.

## Ainéislis *see* Aneslis

## Ainmire *m.*
This name can either be interpreted as meaning 'great lord' or 'wicked lord', as its first syllable can either indicate emphasis or a negative. It was borne by Ainmire Mac Sétnai (d. 569), one of the high kings who ruled from Tara, and by two saints. It has been anglicized as *Anvirre*.

## Airtín *see* Art

### Aisling *f.*

Aislinn means 'a dream, a vision' and is a comparatively recent name, not much used before the nineteenth century. It is often found as *Aislinn* or as the phonetic *Ashling* or *Ashlin*, but has also been recorded in Ireland in the forms *Isleen* and *Elsha*. The name has spread to Britain, no doubt helped by the popularity of similar-sounding, but unrelated, names such as Ashley. In the USA it is usually found in forms such as *Ashlyn* or *Ashlynn* (although Ashlin is also used), indicating a blurring of the boundaries between Aislinn and Ashley. Aisling has been popular in Ireland for several years.

### Alabhaois *see* Aloysius

### Alannah, Alana *f.*

This is usually thought of as the feminine of *Alan*, but it can also be interpreted as coming from the affectionate Irish expression 'alannah' (*a leanbh*), 'O child'. It is moderately popular in the USA, where it is most often spelt *Alanna* and has also developed the form *Alaina* or *Alayna*. *Lana* or *Lanna* are short forms.

### Alaois *see* Aloysius

## Alastar *m.*

This is the Irish form of the Scots name *Alastair*, both being Gaelic forms of the Greek name *Alexander*, 'defender of men'. After his death Alexander the Great became the hero of a wide range of lavish and enormously popular romances which, in the Middle Ages, spread across the world, from India to Iceland. These brought the name to Scotland, where it was given a Gaelic form after Alexander had become a royal name, and from there it spread to Ireland. The name appears in a wide range of forms between the two countries, with spelling such as *Alasdair*, *Alistair*, *Alasdar*, *Alusdar*, and in Ireland, *Alusdrann*. *Alastrina* and *Alastriona* are rarer feminine forms.

## Alayna *see* Alannah

## Albany *m. and f.*

The male and female use of these names has arrived at the same end by different routes. The old Irish word for Scotland was Alba, and Albany was used as a poetic term for either Scotland, or Scotland and England. Both Albany and the related Albion were thought to come from a word meaning 'white' (although language experts now doubt it), and the name Albany was sometimes used to translate the Irish name **Finn**, which means 'white, fair'. As a feminine name Albany is a direct use of the place name, and is an innovation, with strong New Age associations: the singer and ley-line enthusiast Julian Cope, for example, has called his two daughters Avalon and Albany.

## Alby *Ailbhe* m. and f.

The meaning of Alby is not clear, but it probably comes from a word meaning 'white', although it has also been interpreted as 'rock'. It is a very common name in Irish legend and early history. Among the female holders was Ailbhe Grúadhreac ('of the freckled cheeks'), daughter of Cormac Mac Art, mythical High King of Ireland. Described as one of the four best women of her time, she won the love of **Finn** Mac Cool by answering his riddles. By far the most famous male Alby was the sixth-century saint, a contemporary of St **Patrick**, who was converting the south of Ireland at the same time as Patrick was working to the north. Ailbhe was translated Albert, and in the Irish-language press former Taoiseach Albert Reynolds would find his name re-translated to Ailbhe. Nowadays, however, the name is more commonly feminine. It is also found as *Ailbe*, *Alvy*, *Elli* and *Elly*, and for girls *Elva* and *Oilbhe*. (See also **Elvis**.)

### Alexander *see* Alastar

### Alice, Alicia *see* Ailis, Eilis

### Aline *f.*

Aline can be interpreted either as a form of **Eileen** or **Aileen**, or as a separate name from the word *álainn*, 'lovely'.

### Alistair *see* Alastar

### Almha, Almu *see* Alva

### Aloysius *m.*

This name, rare in the rest of the English-speaking world, is comparatively popular in Ireland where it is given in honour of St Aloysius Gonzaga (1568–91), a Spanish nobleman who gave up a glamorous court life to join the Jesuits, the missionary priests of the Counter-Reformation movement, and died after contracting plague from a patient at the hospital where he worked. He was canonized in 1726 and is the patron saint of youth. Aloysius is also found in the short form *Aloys* and in the Irish forms *Alaois* and *Alabhaois*. Aloysius is a form of the name *Louis*, meaning 'famous warrior' and there is a rare feminine form *Aloisia*.

Aloysius was one of the middle names of the writer James Joyce. Another source of the name is as a translation of **Lughaidh**.

## Alusdar, Alusdrann *see* Alastar

## Alva *Almha f.*

The meaning of this name is not known. Alva was one of the Tuatha Dé Danann (see **Dana**) who gave her name, in its old form *Almu*, to the hill and its fortress at Almu in Leinster. The name has sometimes merged into that of *Alma*, which is usually from a Victorian creation celebrating the Battle of Alma (1854) in the Crimean War, although in cases such as Edmund Spenser's *The Faerie Queene*, the name comes from the Latin for 'kind'.

## Alvy *see* Alby

## Amhalgaidh *see* Awley

## Amhlaoibh *see* Auliffe

## Ana *see* Anna Livia

## Andrew *see* Aindrias

### Aneslis *Ainéislis* m.

An old name which probably means 'thoughtful' or 'careful'. It was translated **Standish** or **Stanislaus**, which accounts for the otherwise surprising frequency of this Slavonic name in Ireland. Stanislaus Joyce was the brother of the more famous James Joyce, and it was his support of his brother and family which was largely responsible for James' being able to devote his life to writing.

### Angus, Angustina *see* Aengus

### Annabelle, Annábla *see* Nápla

### Annábla *see* Nápla

### Anna Livia *f.*

This is a name for the literary, qualifying as Irish thanks to James Joyce's *Finnegans Wake*, where Anna Livia Plurabelle is the wife of the hero Humphrey Chimpden Earwicker. On one level of this multi-level novel, the name can be interpreted as a form of *abha life*, the Irish for Dublin's River Liffey; on another, Joyce may have wanted the first part of the name (for Anna Livia also represents Eve) to recall the name *Ana* or

*Anu*, the ancient Irish goddess of abundance and mother of the gods, sometimes described as the Irish Eve, who gave her name to the two mountains in near Killarney known as the Paps of Anu.

## Anne, Anna *see* Áine

## Anu *see* Anna Livia

## Anvirre *see* Ainmire

## Aobnait *see* Eavan

## Aodán *see* Aidan

## Aodh *m.*

This name, which means 'fire', was very common in Ireland in early times, and would originally have been the name of a god. One saint of this name was Aodh or Aed Macbricc (d. 588), a bishop and founder of monasteries who was famed for his skill in medicine, and among its royal bearers Aodh Allán, High King of Ireland between 734 and 743, was an able ruler who extended the influence of the high king over other rulers. There is also the mythical Aodh Eangach who, it was prophesied, would come to rescue the Irish in their time of need, like the Arthur of the

British. Aodh was regularly translated *Hugh*, which accounts for the popularity of that name in Ireland – thus, Hugh O'Neill, Earl of Tyrone (c.1540–1616), and Red Hugh O'Donnell, Earl of Tyrconnell (c.1571–1602), who together led the rebellion against Elizabeth I, would have been Aodhs. The old spelling of the name was *Aed*, and *Aodhaigh* (translated Hughey) is a pet form, while *Ea* is an anglicization. A number of names contain the same first element, or have developed from Aodh: for boys, *Aodhach*, **Aidan**, **Egan** and **Enat**, *Aodhfin*, or *Aodhfionn*, and for girls, *Aodhamair* or *Adamair*.

## Aodhagán, Aodhgan *see* Egan

## Aodhaigh, Aodhamair *see* Aodh

## Aodhan *see* Aidan

## Aodhfin, Aodhfionn *see* Aodh

## Aodhnait *see* Enat

## Aogán *see* Egan

## Aoibheann, Aoibhinn *see* Eavan

## Aoife *f.*

Aoife, which has become one of the most popular

Irish girl's names in recent years, means 'radiant, beautiful', and is one of many names connected with brightness and light given to ancient gods and goddesses. It was held by many legendary and semi-legendary women, and by a daughter of **Dermot**, King of Leinster, who married Strongbow, leader of the Norman invaders of Ireland. Because of the similarity in sound it was translated *Eva*, which accounts for that name's popularity in Ireland. Dermot's daughter often appears in history books as Eva, and Eva Gore Booth (1870–1926), suffragette, peace worker and poet, is a more recent bearer of the name. Eva becomes *Eábha* in Irish, currently popular, along with the form *Ava*.

## Aonghas, Aonghus *see* Aengus

## Ardal *Ardgal*, *Ardghal m.*

This name probably means 'high valour', although it is possible that it belongs with the group of names that come from *art*, 'bear' (see **Art**). It crops up in literature, in the form Arthgallo in Geoffrey of Monmouth's largely fictional *History of the Kings of Britain* of 1136, and in Edmund Spenser's allegorical poem *The Faerie Queene*, where Sir Artegal – the name given a twist so that it can also be interpreted as meaning 'equal to

25

King Arthur' – is the character who represents
Lord Grey of Wilton, Elizabeth I's Lord Deputy in
Ireland who had so cruelly massacred the
Spaniards who came to help the rebelling Irish
in 1580, and whose secretary Spenser had been.
The name was translated Arnold.

### Art *m.*

Art is one of a group of names meaning 'bear',
probably originally used to indicate an outstanding
warrior. The name was borne by a number of
legendary kings, most significantly Art the son of
**Conn** and father of **Cormac**. Although he was a
pagan, legend says that because of the honesty
of his rule two angels hovered over him in battle,
and that he was granted a vision which told him
of the coming of Christianity to Ireland. *Artan*
(*Artán*), *Artigan* (*Artagán*) and *Artin* (*Airtín*) are
all pet forms of the name. Not surprisingly, Art
was translated **Arthur**.

### Arthur *Artúr m.*

Arthur has a long history as a name among Irish
speakers. The earliest surviving record of the
name is of the death in 596 of one Artúr, son of
Aidan Mac Gabráin, king of Dál Riada (western
Scotland and north-eastern Ireland), and the
name is found quite frequently in medieval Irish

history. What is a more difficult question to resolve is the relationship of the famous King Arthur to both this early use of the name among those of Irish descent, and to names such as **Art**. There was a Roman name Artorius (of unknown meaning) and this is usually taken to be the source of Arthur; but as the earliest records of the name are all from the Irish, some would like to interpret King Arthur as not a Welsh-British holder of a Roman name, but as a Northern British hero, one of the Scots who had not yet lost their contacts with their Irish kinsmen. Some have even taken Arthur son of Aidan as the original of the hero. Another connection with the Art names and their meaning of 'bear', is that King Arthur in legend shows many aspects of the ancient Celtic gods, and the bear was an significant sacred animal throughout the vast area of Europe settled by the Celts. Statues and amulets of bears are common through this area and various gods had names containing the element. There was even a bear goddess, Artio, worshipped by the Celts in what is now Switzerland.

**Artigan, Artin** see **Art**

**Artúr** see **Arthur**

**Aryn** *see* **Erin**

**Ashlin, Ashling, Ashlyn, Ashlynn** *see*
**Aislinn**

**Ataigh** *see* **Eochaidh**

**Attracta** *Athracht f.*
St Attracta was a sixth-century virgin saint who
gave her name to Killaraght, Co. Sligo, where she
founded a nunnery. Her feast day is 11 August.

**Atty** *see* **Eochaidh**

**Augusteen** *f.*
This is a particularly Irish feminine form of
the name *Augustine*. It is given in honour of
St Augustine of Hippo (354–430). The boys' names
*Augustine*, or *Ághaistín* and *Aibhistín*, and the old
shortened form *Austin*, or *Oistín*, are common in
Ireland, although not as popular as they were.

**Auley** *see* **Awley**

**Auliffe** *Amhlaoibh m.*
This is the Irish form of the name *Olaf*, 'heir to his
ancestors', which was adopted from the Vikings

who first raided Ireland in 795, and occupied and settled in both Dublin and Waterford in 852. It is also found in the form *Olave*, and was translated *Humphrey*. (See also **Awley** and **Oilibhéar**).

## Aurnia *see* Orla

## Austin *see* Augusteen

## Ava *see* Aoife

## Aveny *see* Eveny

## Awley *Amhalgaidh* m.

Strictly speaking, Awley and its variant *Auley* come from *Amhalgaidh*, an ancient Irish name of unknown meaning, and should not be confused with **Auliffe** from *Amhlaoibh*, but in practice there has long been confusion between the two, both as first and surnames.

## Awnan *see* Adamnan

# b

**Baccán** *see* **Becan**

**Baibín** *f.*

A pet form of *Báirbre*, the Irish form of *Barbara*.
A name from the Greek for 'foreign woman', it was
spread by the fame of St Barbara. She was said to
have been imprisoned by her father, for which he
was punished by death from a lightning bolt,
and became patron saint of those in danger from
lightning (extended to include those in danger
from cannon shot), of architects, engineers, gunners
and firework-makers. Her existence is now in
doubt and the Catholic Church no longer recognises
her feast day. Barbara was used to translate **Gobnet**.

**Bairfhionn, Bairrionn** *see* **Barry**

**Banba** *Banbha f.*

Banba was the name of an early Irish goddesses,

and was also given to the plain where **Tara**, seat of the high kings, lies. The name of this highly important plain came to be used for the whole country, and was another word for **Erin** or Ireland. This poetic term for Ireland was used by the early Irish settlers in Scotland, gave the town of Banff its name, and is still part of the Gaelic vocabulary.

## Banbhan *m.*, Banbhnait *f.*

These names mean 'piglet' and both the masculine and feminine forms were used by early saints. The name comes from the same root as **Banba**.

## Barbara *see* Baibín, Gobnet

## Barclay, Barklay *m.*

These are English forms of the name **Parthalan**. *Berclay* and *Berkley* are also found.

## Barhan *see* Bercan

## Barnaby *m.*

This Hebrew name, a form of the biblical *Barnabas*, was formerly much more common in Ireland, as it was used to translate **Brian**. The shorter form *Barney* was also used. There was an Irish form of the name, *Barnaib*, but this is probably obsolete.

## Barry *Barra, Bairre* m.

This is both a short form of the name **Finbarr**
(or its reverse form, *Bairfhionn* or *Bairrfhionn*)
and a form of **Bearach**, 'pointed, sharp'. Barry has
been enormously popular in the mid-twentieth
century not only in Ireland, but in Britain and
Australia, where it developed the short forms *Baz*
and *Bazza*, and, along with Bruce, became thought
of as a typical Australian name. It is rather out of
favour at the moment in Britain, but still popular
in Ireland and is also being used in the USA. Barry
can also be a Welsh name, when it can either be
from the surname derived from ap Harri ('son of
Harry') or from the place name. (See also **Bercan**.)

## Bartholomew, Bartley, Batt *see* Parthalan

## Baz, Bazza *see* Barry

## Beacán, Beag, Beagóg *see* Becan

## Bean *see* Betha

## Bean Mhí *see* Benvy

## Bean Mhumhan *see* Benvon

## Beanón *see* Benen

**Beanvon** *see* **Benvon**

**Bearach** *m. and f.*
One source of the name **Barry**, Bearach
(*Berach, Berrach*) means 'pointed, sharp', and is
often taken to mean 'spear' or 'sword'. Bearach
was a sixth-century saint who performed many
miracles, including several cases of raising the
dead. (See also **Bercan**.)

**Bearchán** *see* **Bercan**

**Beartlaidh** *see* **Parthalan**

**Beatha, Beathag** *see* **Betha**

**Bébhinn** *see* **Bevin**

**Becan** *Beacán m.*
Becan means 'little man' and began as a pet form
of *Bec*, or *Beag*, (used for both sexes), 'little'. Beag
Mac Dé (d. 553) was a prophet closely associated
with various saints, including **Brendan**, **Kieran** and
*Columba* (see **Colm**). The use of Bec as a female
name is represented by a goddess who, with her
three daughters, guarded a magic well from which
**Finn** Mac Cool won his wisdom. Becan, the name

of a sixth-century saint, in its turn developed a pet form *Beagóg*, and also a variant *Baccán*.

### Bedelia *see* Bidelia

### Béibhinn *see* Bevin

### Benen *Beineón* m.

St **Patrick** gave the name *Benignus* to his favourite follower, who later succeeded him as bishop of Armagh. The name comes from the Latin word meaning 'mild, kind'. Other Irish forms of the names are *Beanón*, *Beineán* and *Bineán*.

### Benvon *Bean Mhumhan* f.

Benvon or *Beanvon* means 'Lady of Munster', and is one of a number of names, including **Benvy**, made up from *bean*, 'lady', plus a place name.

### Benvy *Bean Mhí* f.

This name means 'Lady of Meath'. Meath itself means 'middle (place)', and was the fifth province of Ireland, probably created in the fifth century after a large settlement of people from the north.

### Bercan *Bearchán* m.

Bercan is a pet form of **Bearach**, 'sharp'. St Bercan was a sixth-century saint nicknamed 'the man of two halves' (*fear dá leithe*) because he spent half his life in Scotland and half in Ireland. A renowned prophet, he was much quoted during the wars against the English in Elizabethan times as foretelling an Irish victory. *Bercnan* is a variation of the name and *Barhan* an alternative anglicization.

## Berclay, Berkley *see* Barclay, Parthalan

## Bercnan *see* Bercan

## Bernadette *f.*
The popularity of this name in Ireland is due to affection for St Bernadette Soubirous (1844–79), whose visions of the Virgin Mary at Lourdes led to its becoming the greatest centre of pilgrimage in Europe. The name has also been popular in Australia. *Berneen* is an Irish short form. *Bernadetta* (short form *Detta*) and *Bernadine* are also used.

## Betha *Beatha f.*
This name, and its forms, all mean 'life'. Betha is the Irish form, although it is better known in its Scots Gaelic form *Beathag*, which is also occasionally found in Ireland. Beathag is sometimes spelt *Bethoc*, and anglicized to *Bethia* (otherwise a biblical name meaning 'daughter of Jehovah'). There are also Scots Gaelic masculine

forms, *Beathan* or *Bean*. The Irish and Scots masculine name *Mac Beatha*, 'son of life', meaning a righteous man, is the origin of the name *Macbeth*.

## Bevin *Béibhinn f.*

Bevin means 'white (or fair) lady'. It was the name of both the mother and daughter of **Brian** Boru. A mythical Bevin was a beautiful giantess forcibly betrothed to a giant called **Aodh**. Despite his exceptional beauty, she rejected him and fled to **Finn** Mac Cool for protection, but was later killed by her angry lover, and given an honourable burial by Finn. The name is also spelt *Bébhi(o)nn*, and has been translated *Vivian*. There is another form with Scottish connections, for James Macpherson used a Latinate form, Venina, for the character who plays the role of Béibhinn in his *Ossian* poems.

## Biddy *f.*

This is a pet form of **Brigid**, once so common that it could virtually be used to indicate any Irish woman. However this, plus the development of the unpleasant slang use of the name (as in 'an old biddy') led to a sharp drop in its use, and it is now much rarer. One remarkable holder of the name was Biddy Early (c.1799–1874), a white witch who cured both humans and animals, particularly of eye problems, who imposed and

lifted curses and could see into the future.
Other forms of the name are *Bid* and *Biddle*.

## Bidelia *f.*

Bidelia, or *Bedelia*, is a fanciful form of **Brigid**,
as is the similar *Bidina*. They gave rise to the
short forms *Delia* (already in use as a name from
classical Greece), *Dina* and *Dillie*. These names
are not much used now, as they came to be
thought of as pretentious, but that they were
thought of as typically Irish is seen by the choice
of Delia as the name given to Mrs Malaprop in
his love letters to her by the comic Irishman
Sir Lucius O'Trigger, in Richard Brinsley
Sheridan's play *The Rivals* (1775).

## Bineán *see* Benen

## Birgit, Birgitta *see* Brigid

## Bláthnait *f.*

Bláthnait, *Bláthnaid* or *Blánaid*, meaning 'little
flower, flowerlet', was originally a pet from of
**Bláth**, 'flower'. This, not surprisingly, was
translated *Flora*, with Bláthnait translated *Florence*.
In myth Bláthnait was a married woman who fell
in love with the hero **Cúchulainn** and plotted with
him to elope. She gave the signal to attack her

husband's fortress by pouring milk into a stream that ran from it. Her husband was killed but his bard avenged his death by seizing Bláthnait as she stood at a cliff edge and jumping over, killing them both. In another version of the story her name is given as *Blá(i)thín*, which has the same meaning.

### Blinne *f.*

Blinne is a corruption of *Moninne*, the name of an early Irish saint also known as *Monenna*, **Darerca** and *Bline* (d. c.518). She worked closely with saints **Patrick** and **Brigid**, and founded a nunnery.

### Braden *m.*

This name, from the Irish *bradan*, 'a salmon', has recently been moderately popular in the USA where it also occurs in the versions *Bradon* and *Brayden*. It probably came into use via the surname, rather than as a survival of the old Irish first name from which the surname developed.

### Bradie *see* Brady

### Bradon *see* Braden

### Brady *m.*

This is from an Irish surname, of uncertain meaning. This surname can also be derived from

an English place-name meaning 'broad island'.
It has become moderately popular in the USA,
where the form *Bradie* is also used.

## Bran *m.*

Bran means 'raven'. It is a Celtic name found in
use across the Celtic world, from Ireland in the
west to Greece in the east, where it was the name
of the Celtic chief who sacked the Temple of the
Delphic Oracle in 279 BC. It is the name of a god
in Welsh and Irish tradition, but the best-known
Bran in Ireland is a fictional character who sailed
across the sea to the Isle of Women. After what
seemed a short stay, Bran and his crew returned
to Ireland, only to find that their names had entered
tradition among the descendants of those they
had left behind, and when one sailor leapt ashore,
he turned to dust as if he had been buried for
hundreds of years. The well-known Irish surname
*Branigan* (*Branagán*), is a pet form of Bran,
as is *Brannan* (*Branán*). There is also *Branduff*
(*Brandubh*), 'black raven', which was the name of
both an ancient board game and of a semi-mythical
king of Leinster who died about 605. However,
Bran is far more likely to be given to a dog than a
boy in Ireland today, as it was the name of the
famous wolfhound owned by **Finn** Mac Cool.

## Brandon *m.*

In Ireland this is a form of the name **Brendan**. The mountain in Kerry which is climbed on an annual pilgrimage to celebrate St Brendan's feast day on 16 May is called Mount Brandon. The name can also be from an English surname, which comes from a place-name meaning 'gorse hill'. The name has been enormously popular in the USA, where it also occurs as *Branden*, *Brandin* and *Brandyn*, while the Victorian poet Matthew Arnold used yet another form, *Brandan*, in his poem *St Brandan*.

### Brandubh, Branduff *see* Bran

### Brandyn *see* Brandon

### Branigan, Brannan *see* Bran

### Braon, Braonán *see* Brennan

### Brassal *Breasal m.*

This name, which means 'brave or strong in conflict', was borne by various kings in early Irish lore. It seems somehow to have become associated with cattle, for among its early holders were the fictional High King Brassal Lacking-in-Cattle (Breasal Bó-Dhíobhadh), in whose reign a cattle plague reduced the bovine population of

Ireland to just one of each sex; a king of Leinster called Breasal Beoil who refused to pay cattle tribute to the high king; and a sixth-century prince who stole a cow from a nun. It occurs in the forms *Brasil*, *Brazil*, *Bresal* and *Brissal*, and has a pet form *Breslin* or *Braslin*, or *Breaslán*.

**Brayden** *see* **Braden**

**Brazil** *see* **Brassal**

**Breana** *see* **Bree**

**Bréanainn, Breandán(n)** *see* **Brendan**

**Breann(e), Breanna** *see* **Bree**

**Breasal, Breaslán** *see* **Brassal**

**Bree** *f.*
This is either an independent name from the same root word as, or a short form of the name **Brigid**, from the Irish form *Bríd* or **Bride**. A slightly longer form is *Breeda*, or *Breda*. In the USA the names *Breeanne* and particularly *Breanna* (also *Breeanna*, *Breana*, *Breann*) have become quite popular. These should probably be thought of as a blend of Bree and Anne or Anna, although they shade off

into variants of *Brianne* and **Brianna**, American feminine forms of the Irish name **Brian**, when they take forms such as *Breonna* and *Brieanna*.

## Breege *see* Brigid

## Bren, Brenan *see* Brennan

## Brenda *f.*

Officially Brenda is a name from the Norse *brand*, 'a sword', which became widely known after it was used by Walter Scott in his novel *The Pirate* (1821). However, in Ireland it is used and thought of as a feminine form of the popular boy's name **Brendan**.

## Brendan *Breandán(n)* *m.*

Contact between Wales and Ireland was frequent from the earliest times, and this name began as a Welsh word *breehin*, meaning 'prince'. This was taken into Irish as *Bréanainn*, the modern Irish and anglicized forms of the name coming from Brendanus, the Latin form of the name as used by Irish monks. There are said to be seventeen different St Brendans, two of whom are particularly famous: firstly, St Brendan of Birr (?490–573), known as 'the chief of the prophets of Ireland'. On Brendan's death St *Columba* (see **Colm**) in his monastery on Iona had a vision of angels receiving his soul into heaven; and secondly, St Brendan the Navigator (484–577). The founder of several monasteries, including those of Clonfert and Annadown, he is most famous for the account of *The Navigation of St Brendan*, which tells of his journey across the Atlantic to the earthly paradise of the Land of Promise. This story was so popular in the Middle Ages that it was translated into at least seven languages, as well as surviving in 116 manuscripts of the original Latin. **Brandon** is another version of the name, and in the USA the forms *Brenden* and *Brendon* are also used.

## Brenna *f.*

An American feminine form of the name **Brennan**.

## Brennan *Braonán m.*

The name *Bren* (*Braon*) developed this pet form which has now become the more widely used. Its meaning is not certain, but it probably means 'drop of water' or' tear' and hence, 'sorrow'. Since the earliest records the names **Bran** and *Brannan* and *Bren* and Brennan have regularly been confused, so it is not always possible to tell which is meant. Brennnan has been enjoying moderate success in the USA, where it is also found as *Brenan*, *Brennen*, *Brennon*, *Brennyn* and *Brenon*.

**Breonna** *see* **Bree**

**Bresal, Breslin** *see* **Brassal**

## Brian *m.*

While everyone agrees that Brian is a Celtic
name, authorities are divided as to which Celtic
language has first claim to it, and exactly what
it means; but in any case it seems to come from
a word with the general sense 'high, noble'.
The earlier form of the name in Ireland was
*Brion* (*Brióne*), which later developed into Brian.
However doubtful the history of the name, what
cannot be doubted is the fame of Ireland's
greatest holder of the name, and major factor
in its spread through the world – Brian Boru
(926–1014), High King of Ireland from 1002 until
his death, and national hero and defender of
Ireland against the occupying Norsemen. It was
said that in Brian's reign a single woman, openly
carrying gold, could travel from one end of the
country to the other without being molested. But
Brian's greatest fame was the victorious Battle of
Clontarf, at which, already an old man, he was
killed by one of the fleeing Norsemen. Brian has a
common variant, *Bryan*, and is also found in the
form of the surname *Bryant* or *Briant*. There is an

Irish variant *Brine* and in the USA, where it has recently been very popular, it is also found as *Bryon* and the Spanish-influenced *Briano*.

## Brianna *f.*

Brianna or *Briana* is a modern feminine form of **Brian** that can be found in Ireland, but which has been particularly popular in the USA and Canada. It is also spelt *Bryana* and *Bryanna*. An alternative feminine form, also modern but less frequently found, is *Brianne*, *Briann* or *Bryanne*. These names tend to shade into the *Breeanna* group (see **Bree**).

## Briano, Briant *see* Brian

## Briartach *m.*

This is a Connacht variant of the name **Murtagh**.

## Bride *Bríd f.*

Bride is the usual anglicized Irish form of the name **Brigid**, Ireland's greatest woman saint, while Bríd is the most common Irish form. Bride is technically a pet form but has been so widely used that it should be regarded as an alternative form of the name. It can also be spelt *Bryde*, and pet forms are *Bridie* and *Brídín*. (See also **Bree**, **Bidelia** and **Biddy** for other forms of the name.)

**Bridget, Bridgette, Bridgitte** *see*
**Brigid**

**Bridie, Brídín** *see* **Bride**

**Brieanna** *see* **Bree**

## Brigid *Brighid f.*

Brigid or *Brigit*, which means 'the exalted one',
seems originally to have been a title that could be
given to any goddess, but eventually became the
specific title of a protecting goddess of agriculture
and poetry who was worshipped under slightly
different names in Ireland, Britain and France.
The great St Brigid of Kildare, who died about 523,
seems to have taken over many of the functions
of this goddess in popular culture, for so little is
known about her that some scholars have even
suggested that she never existed. Even this did
not effect her popularity, although out of respect
the name did not come into general use in Ireland
until the eighteenth century. It then became so
popular that it became the typical Irish female
name, particularly in the pet form **Biddy** (see also
**Bree**, **Bidelia** and **Bride**). It also became relatively
popular in other English-speaking countries, where
it was usually anglicized, as in Ireland, to *Bridget*

or *Briget*. This was due to a confusion with the name of St Bridget or *Birgitta*, patron saint of Sweden (whose name was the local form of Brigid), a confusion that would have been helped by the spread of St Birgitta's Order of Bridgettine Nuns. The name has recently been in decline in most of the English-speaking world but has had a modest popularity in the USA where the name also occurs in Scandinavian forms such as *Birgit* (short form *Brit(t)*), Italian forms such as *Brigida*, and Frenchified forms such as *Brigitte*, *Brigett*, *Bridgitte* and *Bridgette*. There is also a short form presently popular in Ireland, *Breege*.

### Brine, Brion, Brióne *see* Brian

### Brissal *see* Brassal

### Brit(t) *see* Brigid

### Brock *Broc* m.
The word 'brock', meaning 'badger', is one of the few words from the British language that entered the English language in Anglo-Saxon times, adopted from the conquered British. The same Celtic root gave the rare early Irish name *Broc(c)*, also meaning 'badger', and both these sources

could give a surname Brock which later became used as a first name. The name, spelt both Brock and *Broc*, is mildly popular in the USA for babies at the moment, while its use in an earlier generation is found in the children's author Brock Cole.

## Brona *f.*, Brone *m.* *Brónach*

Brónach, which means 'sorrowful', could be used in early Middle Ages for either sex, but nowadays is usually found in the rare masculine form Brone, or the more frequent Brona. The actress *Bronagh* Gallagher shows another spelling of the name.

## Brontë *f.*

This surname, belonging to the famous novelist sisters, Charlotte, Emily and Anne, is occasionally used as a first name in their honour. It qualifies as Irish because their father, Patrick, was an Irishman who emigrated to Yorkshire. He changed his surname to Brontë from its original, prosaic Prunty, a surname from the Irish *proinnteach*, meaning 'generous person'.

## Bryan *see* Brian

## Bryana, Bryanna, Bryanne *see* Brianna

**Bryant** *see* **Brian**

**Bryde** *see* **Bride**

**Bryon** *see* **Brian**

**Buagh** *Buadhach, Buach* m.
This name comes from *buaidh*, the Irish word for 'victory', and hence was often translated Victor. From the same Celtic root comes the name of the famous Boudicca or Boadicea, the first-century British queen who led a temporarily successful revolt against the occupying Romans.

# C

**Cabhán** *see* **Cavan**

**Caci** *see* **Casey**

**Cadhan** *see* **Kyne**

**Cadla** *see* **Kiely**

**Caelainn** *see* **Keelin**

**Cahal** *Cathal* m.
Cahal is a phonetic spelling of Cathal, a name made up of the word *cath*, or 'battle' (a common element in early Irish names) and *val*, 'rule'. It is usually interpreted as meaning 'strong in battle' or 'battle-mighty'. It is also found as *Catheld* and *Kathel*. Cathal is the usual form for babies in Ireland at the moment, its use encouraged, it has been suggested, by the fame of Irish Republican soldier and politician Cathal Brugha (1874–1922)

who died in the Civil War, but Cahal is the form that has appeared most in the international media in recent years because of the publicity surrounding Irish Cardinal Cahal Daly. The name was translated Charles, and it is standard to translate Charles back into Irish as Cathal.

## Cahir *Cathaoir* m.

Cahir or *Cathair* is a name made up of two elements, the first, *cath*, a common element in names, meaning 'battle', and the second meaning 'man', so that the name means 'warrior'. Its most famous holder is the legendary High King Cahir Mór ('the Great'), a Leinsterman who ruled until overthrown and killed by **Conn** of the Hundred Battles.

## Cain *see* Kean

## Cainnech *see* Canice

## Cairbre m.

Cáirbre, anglicized as *Carbery*, is a common name in myth and early history. One bearer was a bard, son of Ogma, the god of eloquence and literature, who used the traditional powers of the poet to curse and satirise – bards were supposed to be able to bring on attacks of boils by their satire alone, and even cause death – to help his people in their battles against the evil Fomorians. Another was a son of **Cormac** Mac Art, who succeeded his father as Irish high king and destroyed the traditional royal bodyguard, the Fianna. Yet another was a son of **Niall** of the Nine Hostages and gave his name to Carbury in Co. Kildare.

## Cairenn *see* Niall

## Caisel, Caislín *see* Cashel

## Caisín *see* Cass

## Caít *see* Catriona

## Caitlin *Caitlín f.*

Caitlin or *Caitilín* is an Irish form of Catherine. The Norman invaders of Ireland brought with them an old French variant of Catherine, Cateline, which became popular and developed into Caitlin and its anglicized spelling, **Kathleen**, while the more conventional form of the name became **Catriona**. The name has become enormously popular in the USA, knowledge of it possibly spread by the fame of Caitlin Thomas, writer and wife of the poet Dylan Thomas. The form *Kaitlyn* has recently become the most common spelling in the US, reflecting the way it is pronounced there, as if a blend of Kate and Lyn, rather than with the Irish 'cat' sound. It is also found as *Caitlan*, *Caitlyn(n)*, *Kaitlin*, *Kaitlynn*, *Katelin*, *Katelyn(n)* and *Kaytlin*.

## Caitrín *see* Katrine

## Caitríona *see* Catriona

## Calbhach *see* Calvagh

## Callaghan *Ceallachán* m.

This is a pet form of the name *Ceallach*, a name of disputed meaning (see **Kelly**). Although Callaghan is better known as the surname which came from the first name, the name is also used as a first name. The ancestor of the Callaghans was Callaghan or Ceallachán, King of Munster (d. 952).

## Callum, Calum *see* Colm

## Calvagh *Calbhach* m.

This is a name which was common in the later Middle Ages and means 'bald'. *Calvach* is an alternative spelling. This was the form used by Calvach O'Donnell, chief of Tyrconnell who died in 1566 after being defeated and captured by **Shane** O'Neill, claimant to the kingdom of Ulster.

### Canice *Coinneach, Cainnech* m. *and* f.

Canice, meaning 'pleasant person', was the name of an Irish saint (c.521–598) who was a noted missionary and founder of churches not just in Ireland but also in Wales and Scotland. His name became Canicus in Latin, which gives the anglicized form, and it is also one of the sources of the name **Kenneth**. He is also known as *Kenny*, as shown in the name of his monastery of Killkenny, while in Scotland he has left his name on the Isle of Inchkenneth off Mull, at Kilchennich on Tiree and Kilchainie on South Uist. While usually masculine, Canice has also been used as a female name.

### Cansaidín *see* Consaidín

### Caoilfhionn, Caoilinn *see* Keelin

### Caoilte m.

The meaning of this name has not been satisfactorily explained. In story, Caoilte was **Finn** Mac Cool's cousin and was famous for his speed as a runner.

### Caoimhe *see* Keavy

**Caoimhín** *see* **Kevin**

**Caoinleán** *see* **Quinlan**

**Caolán** *see* **Kelan**

**Caomhán** *see* **Kevin**

**Carbry** *see* **Cairbre**

**Carey** *see* **Cary**

## Carleen *f.*
A particularly Irish feminine form of *Charles*, distinct from the more common forms such as Carla or Caroline. It uses the distinctively Irish affectionate feminine ending, '-een' or '-leen', which has become so popular throughout the English-speaking world in creating new names such as Darleen and Charleen. The form *Carlene* is also found.

## Carmel *f.*
A name given in honour of Our Lady of Mount Carmel. Carmel is a Hebrew word for 'garden' and was the name of a mountain near Haifa in Israel, famous for its lush vegetation and often visited, according to legend, by Mary and the infant Christ.

It was settled by Christian hermits early on, and St *Louis* dedicated a church there to Our Lady of Mount Carmel. Like so many particularly Catholic names, Carmel is found more often in Ireland than in other English-speaking countries.

## Carrick *m.*

A surname either from Ireland or Scotland, both coming from the Celtic word for 'a rock'. The Irish spelling would be *Carraig*. It is more likely to be encountered in the USA than elsewhere.

## Carroll *see* Cearbhall

## Carthage *Carthach m.*

Carthage means 'lover, loving person'. Carthach Mac Saírbrethaig was the ancestor of the widespread MacCarthy family, the commonest 'Mac-' surname in Ireland. As a first name it is also found in the form *Carthy* or *Cartagh*. St Cathage, also known as St Mochta, was a follower of St **Patrick**, and like his leader, British. Legend tells that because he doubted the great ages of the Old Testament patriaụrchs, he had his doubts miraculously disproved by himself living for 300 years.

## Cary *m.*

Carey is a well-established Irish surname with at least eight different sources, including *croidhe*, 'heart', and *ciar*, 'dark, black'. As a first name, Cary or *Carey* is best known from the English actor Cary Grant (1904–86). Born Archibald Leach, his reason for choosing this particular name is not clear. In the USA the spelling *Kary* is also found. However, as a first name it is unlikely to be encountered in Ireland, as it was borne by the informer who betrayed the Invincibles, those responsible for the Phoenix Park murders of 1882, and subsequently became a byword for treachery.

## Cas *see* Cass

## Casey *f. and m.*

Casey derives from the Irish surname which comes from a common early name, *Cathasach*, meaning 'vigilant in war'. As well as being used in Ireland, it has for a time been quite popular in the USA, where the most famous Casey was the folk-hero Casey Jones (1864–1900), an engine-driver whose heroic saving of his passengers at the cost of his own life was immortalized in song. He was actually born Jonathan Luther Jones, his better-known name coming from his home town of

Cayce, Kentucky. His name, however, is always spelt Casey. In the USA the name is currently being used more for girls than boys, with a wide range of alternative spellings, such as *Casy*, *Kacey* and *Kasey* used for both sexes; and the more outlandish *Caci*, *Casie*, *Kacee*, *Kaci(e)* and *Kasey* for girls.

## Cashel *Caisel* m.

This is the Irish place-name used as a first name. It comes from the same root word as the English 'castle', but in Ireland the word refers to a circular stone fort rather than to a fortified noble house. A pet form *Cashlin* (*Caislín*) has also been recorded.

## Casie *see* Casey

## Cass m. *and f.*

Internationally Cass has many sources, mainly as a short form of a name beginning 'Cas-'. For girls it can be short for **Cassidy**, but in Irish Cass or *Cas* is a boy's name meaning 'curly-haired'. *Cassán* is a pet form and *Cassair* an old feminine. *Caisín*, another old form, has been used for both sexes.

## Cassady *see* Cassidy

## Cassán, Cassair *see* Cass

### Cassidy *f.*

This is an Irish surname of unknown meaning which is used as a first name, mainly in the US. Its shortened form *Cassie*, which can also be interpreted as a short form of Cassandra, is even more popular. Cassidy is also found in forms such as *Cassady*, *Cassidee*, *Kassidi* and *Kassidy*; and Cassie as *Cassey*, *Cassi* and *Cassy*.

**Casy** *see* **Casey**

**Cathair** *see* **Cahir**

**Cathal** *see* **Cahal**

**Cathán** *see* **Kane**

**Cathaoir** *see* **Cahir**

**Cathasach** *see* **Casey**

**Catheld** *see* **Cahal**

**Catherine** *see* **Caitlin, Catriona, Kathleen**

**Cathleen** *see* **Kathleen**

## Catriona *Caitríona* f.

This is an Irish form of the name *Catherine*, a name of obscure origin, traditionally interpreted as meaning 'pure'. It was widely used from the early Middle Ages thanks to the popularity of St Catherine of Alexandria. There are a large number of short forms such as *Caít*, *Traoine*, **Triona** and **Riona**, and the name can also be spelt *Catrina* which gives the short form, *Trina*. Catriona is well known as a Scottish name (the original Scots Gaelic form is spelt slightly differently, *Ca(i)triona*), thanks to the success of Robert Louis Stevenson's adventure novel *Catriona* (1893), which made the name much more widely known. (See also **Caitlin**, **Kathleen** and **Katrine**.)

## Cavan *Cabhán* m.

This is the place-name used as a first name. The Irish name for Cavan is An Cabhán, which can mean either a 'hollow', or 'grassy hill'. As both are features of the local geography, it is difficult to tell which is meant at Cavan. Alternatively, it could be a use of the surname which, unusually, is not from the place-name but a form of the surname Keevan, meaning 'having long hair'. It has only been used as a first name fairly recently.

**Caylin** *see* **Keelin**

**Céadach** *see* **Kedagh**

**Ceallach, Ceallachán** *see* **Kelly**

**Ceallachán** *see* **Callaghan**

**Ceallagh** *see* **Kelly**

**Cearbhall** *m.*
Cearbhall was anglicized as *Carroll* and can still
be found in this form (also a common surname),
but the potential confusion with the girl's name
Carol makes it easier to use the Irish form, which
is also spelt *Cearúl(l)*. It was a popular royal name
in the Middle Ages, much used by the Leinster
aristocracy. It later became a favourite name in
the O Daly (Ó Dálaigh) family, and in recent times
has had a distinguished bearer in this tradition in
Cearbhall Ó Dálaigh (1911–77), president of Ireland.

**Cecilia** *see* **Sheila**

**Celsus** *see* **Kelly**

**Ceran** *see* **Kieran**

**Channon** *see* **Shannon**

**Charles** *see* **Manus, Séarlas**

**Charlotte** *see* **Séarlait**

**Chavon, Chevonne, Chivonne** *see* **Siobhan**

**Christie, Christy** *m.*
This Irish form of *Christopher* was made famous by the main character in J. M. Synge's play *The Playboy of the Western World* (1907). Christopher, which means 'bearing Christ', is *Críostóir* in Irish, and the form *Chrystal* (*Criostal*) is also used.

**Cian** *see* **Kean**

**Cianán** *see* **Kenan**

**Ciannait** *see* **Kinnat**

**Ciara** *Ciar f.*
Ciara is a name that seems to have been designed to make life difficult for a writer on first names. Its basic use is as a modern feminine form of **Kieran** (*Ciarán*), meaning 'dark, black', in which case it can also take the forms *Keara*, *Kiera*, *Cieara* and *Ciarra*. As Ciara is the commonest spelling of the girl's name, but the boy's name

is most often spelt with a 'K', these two related names appear widely separated in this book. However, in the USA, where the name is relatively popular, Ciara is also the name of a brand of perfume, and as a first name is more likely to derive from this. Moreover, the perfume is not pronounced as the Irish name is (like 'Kieran' without the 'n'), but as 'see-*are*-a', or identically with another popular American name, Sierra. *Kira* is most likely to be found as an American female equivalent of Kieran. To complicate things further, as Chiara, the Italian form of the name Clare, has become fashionable, the spelling Ciara has been used to represent this name, to emphasise that its first sound is not a 'Ch'. So this name can also represent a pronunciation 'key-*are*-a'. A less confusing alternative for parents to use might be the old Irish feminine of Kieran, *Ciar*.

**Ciaran, Ciarán, Ciarnait** *see* **Kieran**

**Ciarra, Cieara** *see* **Ciara**

**Cillian** *see* **Killian**

**Cináed** *see* **Kenneth**

**Cinnéide** *see* **Kennedy**

**Cionnaodh** *see* **Kenneth**

## Clancy *m.*

This Irish surname comes from the Irish name *Flannchadh*, usually interpreted as 'red warrior' (although this has been doubted by some). It has been used as a boy's name particularly in the USA, but is out of fashion there at the moment. It has also been recorded as a pet form of Clarence.

## Cliona *Clíodhna f.*

Cliona Ceannfhionn ('fair-haired') was the name of a fairy woman particularly associated with Co. Cork. There were many stories of her, in one group of which she figured as a tragic lover, drowned on her way to meet her love; while in others she was a seducer of young men, as well as an inspirer of poets. *Clídna* is the old Irish spelling, and the name has also been recorded as *Cleona* and *Cleana*.

## Clodagh *f.*

This is the name of a river in Co. Tipperary and seems to have been used first in the family of the Marquis of Waterford. Its use has been spread through the fame of Irish singer Clodagh Rogers.

**Coan** *see* **Comgan**

**Cody** *m. and f.*

Cody is an Irish surname which comes from Mac Óda, meaning 'son of Otto', a name that has been in existence since at least the thirteenth century. It is used as a first name, particularly in the USA, where it has become very popular for boys, probably from the fame of the showman Buffalo Bill Cody. It is also used, but less frequently, as a girl's name, when it is usually spelt *Codi*. *Kody* is also used for both sexes, while the feminine form can appear as *Codee*, *Codie*, *Kodee*, *Kodi* and *Kodie*.

**Cóilín** *see* **Colman**

**Coinneach** *see* **Canice**

**Cole** *see* **Comgall**

**Colene** *see* **Colleen**

**Coll** *Colla m.*

This is an early name that means 'high, chief'. It is also used in Scotland, where the three brothers called Coll, the most famous holders of their name in myth, spent some time. These brothers won the kingdom of Oriel (consisting of Armagh, Monaghan and parts of Louth and Tyrone) after a great battle so violent it was said that the spilled blood reached up to the girdles of the warriors.

## Colleen *f.*

From the Irish word *cailín*, meaning 'a girl', this name is popular in Australia and the USA, particularly among families of Irish descent, but is not used in Ireland itself. Its most famous holder is probably the Australian novelist Colleen McCullough. It is sometimes also spelt *Colene* or *Collene*.

## Colm *m.*

This name comes from the Latin word *columba*, 'a dove'. This symbol of peace was a popular choice as a religious name among those turning to the gentler ways of the church from the early Irish warrior society, and there are some thirty-two saints of the name. Its most famous bearer was St *Columba* of Iona (c.521–97), also known as *Colmcille* ('Colm or dove of the Church'), the founder of the great monastery on Iona and apostle of the Scots. The name also occurs as *Colom* or *Colum* (more widely known is the Scottish form *Callum* or *Calum*) and *Columb*, while the name *Malcolm*, primarily Scottish but also used in Ireland, comes from the Gaelic name Mael Coluim, 'follower of St Columba'.

## Colma *see* Colman

## Colman *Colmán* m.

Colman is a form of the Latin name Columbanus, a pet form of **Columba** (see **Colm**), so the name means something like 'little dove'. Colman was a very popular name in early Ireland, and as a consequence there are said to be about 300 Irish saints of this name. These include Colman of Cloyne (c.530–606), a poet and royal bard who converted to Christianity at the age of about 50, and who worked in the Limerick and Cork areas; Colman of Dromore, a sixth-century bishop who worked in Co. Down and Scotland; Colman of Kilmacduagh (d. c.632) who worked in Co. Clare; and Colman of Lindisfarne (d. 676), who was abbot of the monastery there. However, the best-known holder of the name is usually known by its Latin form, as **Columbanus** or **Columban**. He was a Leinsterman who lived from about 543 to 615 but spent much of his working life on the Continent where he founded the monasteries at Luxeuil in the Vosges and Bobbio, famous for its learning, in Italy. He is a popular saint in many countries throughout Europe, and his name is found in various forms in several countries: *Kolman* in the Czech Republic and Slovakia; *Kálmán* in Hungary; *Columbano* in Italy and *Colombain* in France. *Cóilín* is an Irish pet form which is popular in

Connemara. Conductor and pianist Colman Pearce
is a current bearer. Both Columb (see **Colm**) and
Colman were used as girl's names in the past, but
*Colma*, also an old feminine form, is perhaps a
more convenient version to give to girls.

## Colmcille, Colom *see* Colm

## Colombain *see* Colman

## Colum, Columb, Columba *see* Colm

## Columban, Columbano, Columbanus
*see* Colman

## Coman, Cománán *see* Comyn

## Comgall *Comhghall* m.

St Comgall (c.515–602) was abbot of Bangor in
Co. Down whose name is linked with most of
the great saints of the time, but particularly with
*Columba* (see **Colm**), whom he followed to Iona
and on his missionary work in Scotland. He
trained many of the missionaries to pagan
Europe, and many miracles are attributed to him,
depicting him as a great vanquisher of tyranny
and of robbers. The name is also found in the
forms *Cowal* and *Cole*.

## Comgan *Comghán* m.

Comgan may mean 'twin'. St Comgan (also known as *Congan*, *Cowan* and *Coan*) was an eighth-century Leinster chieftain who was driven from power and exiled to Scotland where he founded a monastery at Lochalsh. There are a number of churches dedicated to him in Scotland, and the place-names Kilchoan and Kilcongen, both meaning 'church of St Comgan', refer to him.

## Comhghall *see* Comgall

## Comyn *Cuimín* m.

Comyn comes from *cam*, 'crooked', and would originally have been a nickname. It is also found as *Cummian* and *Cumin*. The name *Coman* (*Comán*) and its feminine, *Comnait*, probably come from the same word.

## Con *see* Conn, Cornelius

## Conaire *see* Connery

## Conall m.

Conall, meaning 'strong as a wolf or hound', is a prominent name in Irish history, held by a number of kings and heroes. These include Conall Cearnach ('the triumphant'), one of the foremost warriors of Ulster and foster-brother to **Cúchulainn**; Conall Corc ('the red'), a fifth-century king of Munster; and Conall Gulban, son of **Niall** of the Nine Hostages (Niall Naoi-ghiallach), who gave his name to the territory of Tyrconnell. Conall Gulban got his name from the great razor-shaped mountain of Benbulben (in Irish, Beann Ghulban) up which, so legend says, he had been made as a boy to run without drawing breath, as part of his training. Conall can also be anglicized as *Connell*, in which case it can be confused with a related name, *Conghal*, 'brave as a wolf or hound', which is also anglicized as Connell.

## Conan *Cónán m.*

This is an old name meaning 'wolf' or 'hound'. It has come to prominence in the past hundred years, firstly from the fame of the author Arthur Conan Doyle who, although born in Edinburgh, was of Irish family. More recently the name has become famous again through Robert E. Howard's fictional creation, Conan the Barbarian, famous through books and film. In these the name is pronounced as in 'cone', rather than with the Irish short 'o' sound. The name is also found as *Conant*.

**Conary** *see* **Connery**

**Conchobarre, Conchobhar, Conchúr**
*see* **Conor**

**Congan** *see* **Comgan**

**Conghal** *see* **Conall**

**Conleth** *Connlaodh* m.
This name, which means 'chief lord', is also found
anglicized as *Conley* and *Conla*, and in Irish as
*Connlao* or *Connlaoi*.

**Conn** m.
There is some debate about what this name
means. Most authorities believe it derives from an
old word that meant 'sense, intelligence' and
which then came to mean 'head, chief'; but it
could also be from the name-element *cu*, meaning
'hound, wolf' and used as a symbol for 'warrior'.
Conn Céad Cathach ('of the Hundred Battles'),
who gave his name to Connacht, would have
lived, if he did exist, some time about 200 AD.
His supposed descendants ruled as high kings of
Ireland until 1022. He is the ancestor of many of
the Irish noble families who kept his name in use,
among them the O'Neills. In the fifteenth and

sixteenth centuries Conn More O'Neill and his son Conn Bacach O'Neill, first Earl of Tyrone, controlled the north of Ireland as loyal supporters of **Garret** More, Earl of Kildare, the effective ruler of the country. The name can also appear as *Con*, and Conn can also be used as a short form of names such as **Conor**. It was translated in the past as *Constantine*, which accounts for the greater use of this name in Ireland than elsewhere. The four Scottish kings called Constantine were also probably Conns.

### Connell *see* Conall

### Conner *see* Conor

### Connery *Conaire* m.

This name probably means 'warrior-lord'. Better known as a surname, Conaire – more properly anglicized as *Conary* – was the name of a mythical king of Tara, known either as Conaire Mór ('the great') or Conaire Caomh ('the gentle'). His motto as king was 'to enquire of wise men so that I myself may be wise', and his reign brought prosperity to his kingdom.

### Connlao, Connlaodh, Connlaoi *see* Conleth

# Conor *Conchobhar* m.

Conor has always been a popular name in
Ireland, even if disguised under its translation of
**Cornelius**. It probably means 'lover of hounds'.
The most famous Conor, usually known as
Conchobhar Mac Nessa, is the king of Ulster in
the stories about Ulster known as The Red Branch
Cycle. He is a mixed character, for he wins his
throne by ruling so well as a temporary ruler that
the people insist he become their permanent king,
yet is universally condemned for his treachery to
**Naoise** and **Deirdre**. A famous bearer is the
academic, politician and writer Conor Cruise
O'Brien. Because of its popularity the name has
developed a range of short forms, including **Con(n)**,
*Naugher*, *Noghor*, *Nohor* and *Conny*, and there is
a modern Irish form of the name, *Conchúr*. In the
USA, where the name is quite popular at the
moment, the alternative spelling *Connor* is the
most popular, and the variant *Conner* is also
found. There is also a feminine form, *Conchobarre*.

# Consaidín m.

This is Irish form of *Constantine*, from the Latin
name Constantinus, 'faithful, loyal', and as such
was felt to be suitable for a cleric. The name is
also spelt *Consaldín* and *Cansaidín* and is a source

of the surname *Considine*. As Constantine is used as a translation of **Conn**, and Consaidín is a direct turning of Constantine into Irish form, it is difficult to tell where one name begins and another ends.

## Constantine *see* **Conn, Consaidín**

## Cooey *see* **Quintin**

## Corey *m. and f.*

Corey is a surname used as a first name. The surname can come either from a Scandinavian or an Irish surname, the latter of which can have several ancestors, including *Gofraidh*, the Irish form of Godfrey. It has been a popular name to give boys in the USA for some time. While Corey is the usual form it is also found as *Corie*, *Corry*, *Cory*, *Korey* and *Kor(r)y*. For girls, the name is usually spelt *Cori*, with other forms such as *Corrie* or *Korri*, and it is not always possible to tell when it should be thought of as this name, or when a form of the name Cora.

## Cormac *m.*

Cormac Mac Art was one of the great legendary high kings of Ireland, the father of **Grania**, who had **Finn** Mac Cool as the leader of his bodyguard, the Fianna. He lost the kingship after his eye was put out in a fight, for the high king had to be unblemished. The meaning of the name is much disputed, but it was popular in early Ireland and has remained well used. A current American bearer is the writer Cormac McCarthy, who shares his name with a twelfth-century king of Leinster.

## Cornelius *m.*

This Roman name is found in Ireland far more than in the rest of the English-speaking world because it was used to translate **Conor**. It is often found shortened to *Corney*, *Con*, *Neilus* or *Neilie*.

## Corrie, Corry, Cory *see* Corey

## Cowal *see* Comgall

## Cowan *see* Comgan

## Crevan *Criomhthann m.*

This name, popular in early times but now uncommon, means 'fox'. It is said to have been St *Columba*'s name (see **Colm**) before he entered the Church. Now it is better known as a surname, as in the writer Tomás Ó Creomhthann, author of *The Islandman*.

## Criostal, Críostóir *see* Christie

## Cronan *Crónán* m.

Cronan comes from the word *crón*, 'dark skinned, sallow', and is the name of a number of saints. It is also found in the forms *Croney* and *Cronin*. St Cronan of Roscrea was a seventh-century monk who was so concerned to give shelter to those in need that he moved his monastery to the roadside after a group of night-time travellers failed to find it because it was sited too far off the beaten track.

## Cuan *Cuán* m.

This is virtually the same name as **Conan**, both being pet forms of *cu*, meaning 'hound' and, in earlier times, 'wolf'. This was a common element in fighters' names, and had more or less the force of 'warrior'. It is one of the early Irish names that has been revived in the twentieth century.

## Cúchulainn m.

Cúchulainn was the greatest of all the Irish heroes, the man who defended Ulster single-handedly against the invading forces of Connacht. He won his name 'Hound of Culann' when, as a mere boy, he killed the fierce beast who guarded Culann's fortress when it tried to stop him entering at night. To make up for having killed Culann's guard-dog he offered to protect the property himself, and thus got his name.

## Cuimín, Cumin, Cummian *see* Comyn

## Cúmhái, Cú Mhaighe *see* Quintin

**Dabacc, Dabag, Dabhag** see **Dáibhí**

**Dagda, Daghda** see **Dáire**

**Dahy** see **Dáithí**

**Dáibhí** *m.*
This is the Irish form of Davy, and the commonest form of the name *David* used in Irish. The full form of David in Irish is *Daibhead* (sometimes found as *Daibhéid* or *Davet*), and there are old pet forms, *Dabacc*, *Dabag* and *Dabhag*.

**Daimhín** see **Davin**

**Dáire** *m.*
Dáire means 'the fruitful one', and may well have been an alternative name for the *Dagda* (*Daghda*), 'the good or effective god', the ancestor god of

the Irish people. It is a very early Irish name and occurs in a number of different stories about apparently different people, but they probably all come from the same original, or are in some way connected. It early times it was also used as a female name, but it is unlikely to be used for girls today. It was anglicized to *Dary*. (See also **Darina**.)

### Dáirine *see* **Darina**

### Dairinn *see* **Dorean**

### Dáithí *m.*

Dáithí, anglicized *Dahy*, started life as the name *Nathí* or *Naithí* (anglicized as *Nathy*), meaning 'nephew of Eo', which can be further interpreted as 'nephew of a tree' (a tree being a symbol of a champion). However, the name was reinterpreted in the Middle Ages as a short form of the word *daithe*, meaning 'swiftness', or 'the swift one', and got its current form. There was a real king of this name who died in 445, but many of the overseas adventures he is said to have had could not have happened literally. However, he does seem to have been a successful war-leader, who led his troops on raids in Britain. His grave, marked by a red pillar-stone, is still to be seen today at

Rathcroghan, Co. Roscommon. The name is also found as **Dathy**, and sometimes interpreted as a form of **Daibhead** (see **Dáibhí**).

## Daley *Dálach* m.

Daley or *Daly* is the surname used as a first name. The surname in turn came from the name *Dálach* which meant 'someone who often goes to gatherings', so would have started out as a nickname. Its use is by no means confined to the Irish, as shown by the athlete Daley Thompson.

## Dallan *Dallán* m.

This name means 'blind one' and was quite widely used in the past. A famous holder was the late-sixth-century poet Dallán Forfaill, called the chief poet of Ireland, who composed a celebrated hymn to St **Columba** (see **Colm**). His name was really a nickname, for Dallán Forfaill means 'the blind man of eloquence'. The name is still in use, especially in the parish of Kildallon, Co. Cavan, which gets its name from St Dallan.

## Dalton m.

This is a surname which is currently very fashionable as a first name in the USA. It can have two sources: from several English place-names meaning 'settlement in the valley'; or from a Norman surname, originally d'Autun, 'from Autun', a French place-name meaning 'fort of Augustus'. After a branch of this Norman family settled in Co. Clare Dalton became a well-known Irish surname.

## Daly *see* Daley

## Damhán *see* Davin

## Damhnait, Damhnat *see* Devnet

## Dana *f.*

Dana or *Danu* was a goddess who gave her name to the main group of other-world beings in Irish mythology, the Tuatha Dé Danann, 'the people of the goddess Danu'. She is rather a shadowy figure, who was early on identified with the goddess *Anu* or *Ana* (see **Anna Livia**), and seems to be a mother goddess. She is also probably connected with a Celtic river goddess with a similar-sounding name who gave her name to rivers from India to Britain, including the Danube and the Welsh Don. However, not all uses of Dana as a first name come from her. The well-known Northern Irish singer Dana traces her name to the Irish word *dána*, 'bold'. As a male name, as in the comic actor Dana Carvey, Dana comes from a

Germanic surname meaning 'a Dane', and some feminine uses of the name in the USA, where it is quite popular at the moment, may be from the same source.

## Dara *m. and f.*

This is a short form of *Mac Dara*, 'son of the oak', and was the name of a Connemara saint, the patron of the local fishermen. From there it spread to the rest of Ireland, where it is now quite popular. *Darach* (in Scotland *Darroch*) is an alternative form. The surname *Darragh* (occasionally *Daragh*), a popular first name, comes either from this or the related name *Dubhdara*,'black oak'. Although mainly a boy's name, Dara is now used occasionally for girls, probably encouraged by the fact that most European names ending in 'a' are feminine.

## Darby *m.*

Darby or *Derby* was at one time a common name in Ireland, and is still found today. It is usually a surname from the English place-name Derby, used as a first name, but in Ireland it was a standard translation of **Dermot**.

## Darcy *m. and f.*

Usually, Darcy is described as a surname

originally given to someone from (*de*) the French place called Arcy – hence, d'Arcy. However, in Ireland the surname comes from an anglicization of O Dorchaidhe, 'descendant of the dark one'. Once exclusively male, Darcy is now well-used for women, especially in the USA. Feminine use is especially well-represented in the world of ballet, in the names of *Darcey* Bussell and *Darci* Kistler. Other spellings are *Darcie* and *D'Arcy*.

### Dareen *see* Darina

### Daren *see* Darren

### Darerca *f.*
Darerca, which means 'daughter of Erc' (Erc could mean either 'speckled' or 'salmon'), is a name with strong religious associations. As well as being the name of the saint also known as **Blinne** and of at least one other saint, it is also said to have been the name of St **Patrick**'s sister (the mother of seventeen bishops) and of St **Kieran**'s mother.

### Darin *see* Darren

### Darina *Dáiríne f.*
This name is probably a feminine form of **Dáire**. In myth, Darina or *Dareen* was a daughter of the

High King **Tuathal**. She was bigamously married to a king of Leinster after he had claimed that his first wife, her elder sister, had died. When the sisters found out the truth they died of shame. The revenge extracted for the insult was a tribute, the paying of which was a cause of war between the high kings and Leinster for generations.

## Darragh *see* Dara

## Darren *m.*

The origin of the name Darren is rather obscure, but the most likely source is from the Irish surname, a version of *Darragh* (see **Dara**). Its growth as a first name occurred in America, where the first prominent user was an actor called Darren McGavin (b. 1922), although it became more popular in the 1960s as a result of the successful TV series *Bewitched* and the fame of singer Bobby Darin. It was well used throughout the English-speaking world in the '60s and '70s, and is enjoying a revival in the USA today. It is also spelt *Daren*, *Darin*, *Darran*, *Darrin*, *Darron* and *Derron*, and there is a feminine form, *Darrene*.

## Dary *see* Dáire

**Dathy** *see* **Dáithí**

**Davan** *see* **Davin**

**Davet, David, Davy** *see* **Dáibhí**

**Davin** *Damhán, Daimhín m.*
Davin is an anglicization of two related Irish
first names, Daimhín and Dámhan. Daimhín
means 'deer' or 'ox', and is also the source of the
surnames *Devin* and Devine, while Damhán means
'little ox' or 'stag', and can also be anglicized as
*Davan*. In modern Irish the words mean only 'ox'
and 'little ox', having lost the connection with
'deer'. The girl's name Davina, a Scottish form
of *David*, is not connected with Davin, but there
is no reason why it should not be used as a
feminine form of Davin if parents choose.

**Davnit** *see* **Devnet**

**Deaglán** *see* **Declan**

**Deamán** *see* **Dermot**

**Dearbhail, Dearbhaile, Dearbhla** *see*
**Dervla**

## Dearbhorgaill *see* Ciernan

## Deasún *see* Desmond

## Declan *Deaglán m.*

St Declan is said to have been preaching in
the south of Ireland even before the arrival of
St **Patrick**. He founded the monastery in Ardmore,
Co. Waterford, and is still an important figure in
local lore. On the beach at Ardmore, for instance,
is a rock known as St Declan's Rock on which
St Declan's bell was floated back to him after it
had been left on the shore of France by a careless
follower as they returned from a visit to Rome.
This rock sits on two others, creating a narrow
passage below through which people crawl in the
hope of a miraculous cure. Declan has been a
very popular name in the twentieth century, and
there is a modern feminine form, *Decla*.

## Deirbhile *see* Dervla

## Deirdre *f.*

The meaning of this name is not clear, but is often
given as 'chatterer'. However, its popularity is due
not to its meaning but to the tragic story of Deirdre,
one of the most famous and frequently re-told

tales from early Ireland. Deirdre was the most beautiful woman of her time, but it was prophesied that she would cause much slaughter. Nevertheless the king, **Conchobhar** Mac Nessa (see **Conor**), decided to marry her. Deirdre, however, preferred the handsome young **Naoise** to the old king, and they eloped to Scotland. After some time they were offered a safe conduct back to Ulster, but Conchobhar treacherously had Naoise murdered, and forced Deirdre to live with him. After a year he announced that he was passing her on to the man who had killed her lover, unable to bear more suffering, Deirdre dashed her brains out against a rock. The story was used by the writers of the Irish revival, including W. B. Yeats (*Deirdre*, 1907) and J. M. Synge (*Deirdre of the Sorrows*, 1910), and this led to extensive use of the name. By the 1920s it had spread to the rest of the English-speaking world. It is occasionally met with in its old Irish spelling *Derdriu*, but the standard Irish spelling, or the form *Deidre*, are by far the commonest, except in the USA where *Deidra* is the form most likely to be given to a baby. There can also be found the forms *De(e)dra*, *Deidre*, *Diedra*, and the short form *Dee* can also be *Deigh*. Other attempts to master the Irish spelling have resulted in *Deidrie*, *Dierdrie* and *Derdre*.

**Delia** *see* **Bidelia**

**Delma** *see* **Fidelma**

**Deman, Demitrius** *see* **Dermot**

**Deoradhán** *see* **Doran**

**Derby** *see* **Darby, Dermot**

**Derdre, Derdriu** *see* **Deirdre**

**Derinn** *see* **Dorean**

**Dermot** *Diarmaid* m.

Dermot has been a very popular name in Ireland throughout the ages and was borne by several early kings and a number of saints. In story, the most famous Dermot was the one who eloped with **Grania**. She had been betrothed to **Finn** Mac Cool in his old age, but preferred the famously handsome Dermot. The lovers spent sixteen years as fugitives from Finn's revenge, but eventually, with the help of **Aengus** Og, the god of love, they were allowed to settle together. At a hunt held to celebrate the reconciliation, however, Finn encouraged Dermot to tackle a magic boar, and then allowed him to die of his wounds. Not surprisingly for such a popular name in all regions of Ireland, it has several variations: *Diarmuid*,

*Diarmid*, *Diarmait*, *Diarmod* and a Scottish Gaelic form, *Diarmad* or *Diarmid*. Anglicized versions include *Dermid*, *Dermod* and **Kermit**, and it has been translated **Darby** and *Derby*, *Derry*, *Demitrius* and most often as **Jerome** or **Jeremiah**. An early Irish pet form was *Deman* (*Deamán*).

### Derron *see* Darren

### Derry *see* Dermot

### Derval, Dervila, Dervilia *see* Dervla

### Dervin *see* Dorean

### Dervla *Dearbhail f.*

When discussing this name, writers on Irish first names do not seem able to agree on which two similar Irish names give which similar anglicizations. Of the Irish names, the most popular at the moment is *Dearbhail*, usually explained as meaning 'true desire'. This name is anglicized as Dervla, *Derval* and *Dervilia*. The other is *Deirbhile*, 'daughter of a poet', also given as a source of Dervla, and of *Dervila*. It is not surprising then, that some parents looking for an Irish form of Dervla have opted for re-spelling it in Irish as *Dearbhla*, or that forms half-way between the two Irish names appear, such as *Dearbhaile*.

Dervla Murphy, the travel writer, has brought the name to a wider audience.

### Dervorgilla *see* Tiernan

### DeShawn *see* Shawn

### Desmond *Deasún* m.

Desmond is one of those Irish names that have become so naturalized in the names of the English-speaking world that it is hardly thought of as Irish any more, and indeed, the form Deasún is a translation of the English name into Irish. However, Desmond is Irish, and means 'a man from Desmond (south Munster)'. Its use as a first name probably came from the title of the Earls of Desmond, many of whom played an important part in Irish history. There is an older Irish form of the name, **Desmumhnach**, which was the source of the surname. Desmond is shortened to *Des* or *Desy* (or *Dez* and *Dezzi*) and in the USA is also found spelt *Dezmond*.

### Detta *see* Bernadette

### Devin *see* Davin

### Devnet *Damhnait* f.

This name means 'fawn' and occurs in two

different forms, associated with two different saints. One, also known as *Damhnat*, is associated with Tedavnet, Co. Monaghan, and her crosier is preserved in the National Museum, Dublin. The other is St *Dympna* of Gheel in Belgium, where her relics are preserved. The story of Dympna (also found as *Dymphna* and more rarely *Dimpna*) belongs to fiction rather than fact. She is said to have been a Celtic princess (the only reason for treating her name as a form of Damhnait) who fled to Belgium to escape her father's incestuous attentions, and was murdered there by him. This act of insanity on his part, and the cures of the mentally sick accompanying her beatification, led to her becoming the patron saint of the insane, and a number of mental hospitals in Belgium and the USA bear her name. Devnet is also found as *Davnit* or *Downet*.

**DeWayne** *see* **Duane**

**Dez, Dezmond, Dezzi** *see* **Desmond**

**Diarmad, Diarmaid, Diarmait, Diarmid, Diarmod, Diarmuid** *see* **Dermot**

**Diedra, Dierdrie** *see* **Deirdre**

**Dillie, Dina** *see* **Bidelia**

**Dimpna** *see* **Devnet**

**Doireann** *see* **Dorean**

### Dolan *m.*
This is the Irish surname, of disputed meaning, used as a first name.

### Dolores *f.*
Originally a Spanish name from a title of the Virgin Mary, Maria de los Dolores ('of the Sorrows'), this has been adopted by devout Catholics. It is well used in Ireland where one holder is Dolores O'Riordan, lead singer with The Cranberries group.

**Domhnall** *see* **Donal**

### Donagh *Donncha, Donnchadh m.*
Donagh or *Donough* probably means 'brown warrior' and is the Irish equivalent of the Scottish *Duncan*. Donagh is a name that crops up throughout Irish history. It was given to a son of **Brian** Boru; a Donagh O'Brien was king of Thomond in the thirteenth century; and another of the same name was earl of Thomond in seventeenth century.

The name is also spelt **Donogh** or **Donnacha** and has been anglicized as **Donaghy**. Any Irishman called Dionysius, Donat or Donatus was probably originally a Donagh, as these, along with Denis, were used to translate the name.

## Donal *Dónal, Domhnall* m.

Donal or **Donall** means 'world-mighty'. The name has been used steadily through the ages, and in the ninth century was regarded as a royal name. *Dónal Óg* ('Young Donal') is the title of a fifteenth-century love song, versions of which are found not only in Ireland and Scotland, but in North America, Australia and wherever the Gaels went. By the seventeenth it was so common that it became a general term for an Irishman, and today the pet form **Donie** is used for a country bumpkin in the Cork area. The name was taken by the Scots to Scotland, and St Donal, better known by the Scottish form of the name **Donald**, was a Scot who died in the early eighth century. After the death of his wife, he had retired to lead a religious life with his nine daughters, who are generally known as the Nine Maidens. There is a rare feminine form, **Donelle**.

## Donavan, Donavon *see* Donovan

## Donegal *m.*

This Irish place-name, which comes from the Irish Dún na nGall, 'fort of the foreigners,' is on record as a first name. The foreigners referred to are the Vikings, who took over a fort in the area in the tenth century.

## Donegan *Donnagán m.*

This is the surname used as a first name. The surname in turn comes from Ó Donnagáin, 'descendant of Donnagán', an old name which was a pet form of the name *Donn*. This name can be interpreted as meaning 'brown, dun' and was the name of an important god, the king of the dead.

## Donelle, Donie *see* Donal

## Donla *Dúnlaith f.*

This is a name which occurs quite often in royal genealogies and which was revived in the twentieth century. It can be interpreted either as 'lady of the fortress' or 'brown lady'. It can also be anglicized as *Dunla* and spelt *Dunfhlaith* in Irish.

## Donn *see* Donegan

## Donnabhán *see* Donovan

### Donnagán *see* Donegan

### Donncha, Donnchadh, Donogh, Donough *see* Donagh

### Donovan *Donnabhán* m.
This is an old Irish first name, meaning 'dark brown (person)', which became a surname. Its spread as a first name owes much to the fame of the Scottish-born singer Donovan Leich (usually known simply by his first name). In the USA, where the name is moderately popular, it is also found as *Donavan* and *Donavon*.

### Doraine *see* Dorean

### Doran m.
Doran or *Dorran* is a surname meaning '(descendant of) *Deoradhán*', itself an old first name meaning 'exiled person'. Doran is being used increasingly as a first name.

### Dorean *Doireann f.*
Traditionally interpreted as meaning 'sullen', this name is now thought to be a version of the name *Dairinn* (earlier Der Finn), 'daughter of Finn', which is anglicized as *Dervin* or *Derinn*. *Doreen* is often described as a version of Dorothy rather

than of Dorean, or at best possibly influenced by it, but it is much more likely that Doreen, with its typically Irish '-een' ending, is a version of Dorean, particularly as Doreen was introduced as a name to the public in 1894 in a novel of the same name by Edna Lyle. Lyle had already used an Irish name for another title in 1882 when she published *Donovan*. Dorean is also found as **Dorren**, and the rare names **Doraine** and **Dorinne** are probably other versions of it. Both Doreen and Dorean were popular in Ireland in the twentieth century.

**Dorran** *see* **Doran**

**Dorren** *see* **Dorean**

**Dorrie** *see* **Fardoragh**

### Dougal *Dubhghall* m.

Dougal or *Dugald*, meaning 'dark stranger', was a name the Irish gave to the invading Vikings, and is traditionally said to have been used of the darker Danes, while the fairer Icelanders and Norwegians had the term *Fingal* ('fair stranger') applied to them. As a first name, Fingal is primarily Scottish (although it is also the name of an Irish earldom), but Dougal is used as a first name in both countries. It is also found in the forms *Dúghall* and *Dugal*. Like so many early invaders and settlers, the Vikings were soon absorbed into the local population and the name quickly lost any suggestion that its holders were not Irish.

### Downet *see* **Devnet**

### Doyle *m.*
This is the Irish surname used as a first name. The surname comes from Ó Dubhghaill, 'descendant of **Dougal**'.

### Duald *Dubhaltach m.*
This name means 'black jointed', which may indicate 'dark limbed'. It can also be spelt *Dualtach* and anglicized as *Dualtagh*.

### Duana *m. and f.*
A modern name from the Irish *duan*, 'poem, song'.

### Duane *Dubhán m.*
This is an American name taken from an Irish surname, which comes in its turn from the first name *Dubhán*, 'dark(-haired) person'. It came into general use in the 1950s thanks to the fame of the singer Duane Eddy, and became popular throughout the English-speaking world. It is also spelt *Dwane* and *Dwayne* (the commonest form in

the USA) and can also be found as *Dwain*, *Dwaine* and, particularly among US blacks, *DeWayne*.

## Dubhaltach *see* Duald

## Dubhán *see* Duane

## Dubhdara *see* Dara

## Dubhghall *see* Dougal

## Duff *m.*

Duff is another surname used as a first name in both Ireland and Scotland. It comes from the word *dubh*, 'black', which would either have been a short form of one of the many names starting with this element (see for example **Dougal**, **Duald**, **Duane**), or a nickname for a dark person.

## Dugal, Dúghall *see* Dougal

## Duibheasa *see* Una

## Duncan *see* Donagh

## Dunla, Dúnlaith *see* Donla

## Dwain, Dwaine, Dwane, Dwayne *see* Duane

**Dwyer** *m.*
The Irish surname, which comes from elements meaning 'black' and 'dun-coloured', probably owes its occasional use as a first name to the fame of United Irishman Michael Dwyer (1771–1815), who led the 1798 rising in Wicklow against the English. He was a daring and resourceful guerrilla leader who became a popular hero and there is a whole body of folklore about his hair's-breadth escapes from English soldiers.

**Dymphna, Dympna** *see* **Devnet**

# e

**Ea** *see* **Aodh**

**Eábha** *see* **Aoife**

**Eachann** *m.*

Eachann is usually interpreted as a form of the name *Eachdhonn*, made up of the words *each*, 'horse', and *donn*, 'lord'. As such it would fit in with a number of early Irish names containing the word *each*, such as the male names *Eachdha* or *Eacha*, meaning either 'horse-like' or 'horse-god' and the female *Eachna*, in legend both beautiful and one of the cleverest women in the world. But it has recently been suggested that Eachann is actually an Irish form of the Scandinavian name Hakon, borrowed from the Vikings. Hakon can derive either from an element meaning 'horse', or one meaning 'high' plus an element meaning 'descendant'. Eachann was taken by the Scots

to Scotland, where it is still in use. There it was
thought of it as having the sense 'horse-lord', as it
was translated *Hector* (the source of this relatively
common Scots name), not just because of a vague
resemblance in sound, but because the Trojan hero
Hector had a reputation as a mighty horseman.

## Éadaoin *see* Étain

## Ealga *f.*
An unusual name, Ealga, meaning 'noble',
belongs with the group of names like **Erin** and
**Banba** which come from terms for Ireland. In this
case the source is the Inis Ealga, the 'Noble Island',
a poetic term for Ireland.

## Eamhair *see* Emer

## Eamon *Éamonn* m.
The Irish form of the English name *Edmund*,
meaning 'rich protection'. It was very popular,
spelt equally often *Eamonn*, although this form
is perhaps slightly the more common among
older people. Its most famous recent bearer
was the politician Éamon de Valera (1882–1975),
born in the USA (a fact that saved his life when
condemned to death by the British for his part in
the 1916 Easter Rising) to an Irish mother and

Cuban father. He was president of Ireland from 1959 to 1973.

### Éanán *see* Enan

### Éanna *see* Enda

### Earc *see* Murry

### Earnán *see* Ernan

### Eavan *Aoibhinn* f.

Aoibhinn or *Aoibheann* means 'beautiful radiance'. It was used in the tenth century for a number of princesses, and was revived in the twentieth century, notably in the poet Eavan Ashling Boland. *Eavnat* (*Aobnait*) is a related name meaning 'radiant girl'.

### Edan, Edana *see* Aidan

### Edmund *see* Eamon

### Edna f.

This is probably best thought of as an Irish name. Although it is the name of Enoch's wife in the biblical *Apocrypha*, this is an obscure source and it is far more likely that its general use comes from an anglicization of **Eithne**. It was one of a number of Irish names popular in Britain in the first thirty years of the twentieth century, but it now seems to be generally out of fashion. As many of the names from this period are becoming popular once more, however, it may be due for a revival.

## Eenis *see* Aengus

## Egan Aogán *m.*

Egan is a pet form of **Aidan**, 'little fire'. Its Irish form is also spelt *Aodhgan* and *Aodhagán*. Egan O'Rahilly (Aogán Ó Rathaille, c.1670–1729) was the outstanding poet of his age. He specialized in the vision-poem or aisling (see **Aislinn**), in which he told of prophesies of other-world women that Ireland would triumph over her enemies. In folklore he is shown as a wise trickster, always ready with a witty verse, and in one story even gets the better of Dean Jonathan Swift, the author of *Gulliver's Travels*. *Iagan* is the name's Scottish form.

## Éibhear *m.*

Éibhear was one of the mythical leaders of the first Gaelic settlers in Ireland. He and his brother *Éireamhóin* or *Eireamhón* (anglicized as *Erevan*, *Heremon* or *Hermon*) were the sons of Míl or Milesius (from whom the settlers, the Milesians, took their name). They led the true Gaels who

were to win the country from the Tuatha Dé
Danann (see **Dana**). But the whole family is a
scholarly invention to provide sources for the
names of Ireland. So the name of Éibhear's father
(also given as Míle Easpain) means 'soldier of
Spain', from where the Irish Celts were thought
to have come (indeed, archaeologists have shown
links between the Celts in Spain and some of
those who settled in Ireland); their mother was
called Scota, or 'Irishwoman' in Latin; his
brother's name, Éireamhóin, is based on Ériu,
the old form of the name Eire; and Éibhear itself
comes from Eberus, an Irish form of the Latin
Hibernus, 'Irishman', via its old form, Éber. Éibhear
was well used into the nineteenth century and has
recently had a revival. It has been translated
Harry, Ivor and most often *Heber*, an otherwise
rare biblical name, and anglicized as *Ever*.

### Éibhleann *see* Evelyn

### Eibhlín *see* Aileen, Eileen, Evelyn

### Éigneachán *see* Eneas

### Eileanóir, Eiléanór, Eilíonóra *see* Lean

### Eileen *Eibhlín f.*

The conquering Normans brought with them to

Ireland the name Aveline or Avelina as part
of their own inheritance from their Germanic
ancestors. The meaning of the name is obscure,
but it may mean 'wished-for child'. In Irish
Aveline became *Aibhílín* and *Eibhlín* (which can
be pronounced with or without a 'v' sound in the
middle). These in turn were anglicized as Eileen,
**Aileen** or **Evelyn**. Eileen is shortened to *Eily* and
in Ireland can also be anglicized as *Ella*, *Ellen* or
*Ellie*, and was translated Helen. Indeed, some
Irish people regard Eileen as an Irish version of
Helen. *Ilene* is a spelling most often found in
America. The name was very popular in the first
part of the twentieth century in Ireland, and in
Britain in the 1920s and '30s, but is rather out of
favour now, Aileen superseding it in popularity.
It is still quietly used in the USA.

## Eilis *Eilís f.*

Strictly speaking, Eilis is a form of *Elizabeth* and
**Ailis** a form of *Alice*. But in practice it is doubtful if
users make the same clear distinction that books
on names do, particularly when other pairs of
names, like **Aileen** and **Eileen**, are simply different
spellings of the same name. The confusion seems
to be long-standing, as Eilis was translated in the
past as both Elizabeth and Alice. It is also found

in the anglicized forms *Eilish* and *Eillish*. Elizabeth is a biblical name meaning 'God is my oath'. Used in honour of Elizabeth or Elisabeth, cousin of the Virgin Mary and mother of John the Baptist, it is found in various forms across the Christian world.

## Eily *see* Eileen

## Eimear, Éimhear *see* Emer

## Éimhín *see* Evin

## Einín *f.*
Einín is a modern name which comes from *éan*, 'bird', and so can be translated 'little bird'.

## Éire *see* Erin

## Éireamhóin, Éireamhón *see* Éibhear

## Eireen *f.*
This unusual modern name, found in both Ireland and Britain, can be interpreted as either a blend of Irene and **Eileen**, or as a play on 'Eire' combined with the Irish feminine ending '-een'.

## Eirnín *see* Ernan

## Eithne *f.*

In the charming fourteenth-century story, the beautiful Eithne was one of the Tuatha Dé Danann (see **Dana**). At one point she suddenly refused all food, taking only the milk of two cows from 'the righteous land of India'. The sea-god Manannán, who knew the cure for all illness, diagnosed that her guardian demon had left her and been replaced by a guardian angel, and that she was no longer one of the Tuatha Dé Danann, but a Christian. Eithne was a very popular name in early times in royal and religious circles, and there are nine saints of the name, one of them also known as *Ethenia*. It can be found in the forms *Etna*, *Ethna*, *Etney* and occasionally *Ethni*, while the singer *Enya* reflects another pronunciation. Anglicized versions have given the names **Edna** and **Ena**. Eithne was revived in the twentieth century, one famous holder being the actress Eithne Dunne (1917–88).

## Elizabeth *see* Eilis

## Ella, Ellen, Ellie *see* Eileen

## Elli, Elly *see* Alby

## Elsha *see* Aislinn

## Elva *see* Alby

## Elvis *m.*

Is Elvis an Irish name? There is of course only one immediate source of the name, Elvis Presley. But there has been much debate as to where *his* name came from. It was recorded as a rare name in the USA before it shot to fame, and was also Elvis Presley's father's middle name. As Southerners, his family were part of a society with a tradition of making up names, or making new names by blending two names together, such as Ellis and Alvin, and this may have been its source. On the other hand, the family was ultimately of Irish descent, and an Irish connection with the name does exist. The only other recorded source of the name Elvis is in the Welsh place-name St Elvis in Pembrokeshire, but this should perhaps more properly be written 'St Elvi's', as it refers to the Irish St **Alby** who is said to have baptized St *David*, the patron saint of Wales. Bearing in mind that Alby as a feminine name is often spelt Elva, Alby must be a strong candidate for the original of Elvis.

## Emer *f.*

Emer was the wife of **Cúchulainn**. The saga's description gives an impression of the old ideal of an Irishwoman, for she was said to have 'the six gifts of womanhood – ... beauty, ... chastity, ... sweet speech, ... needlework, ... voice and ... wisdom'. Her father opposed the match and Cúchulainn, who had fallen in love at first sight, fought hard to win her. But he was not faithful, and when he had an affair with *Fand*, wife of the sea god Manannán, the jealous Emer decided to murder her rival. She found the two lovers together, but when she saw how Fand loved Cúchulainn, Emer, from her great love, offered to give him up for the greater good. Fand, realising the strength of Emer's love, offered to go back to her husband, and with the help of a draught of forgetfulness marital harmony was restored. The name, currently most popular as *Eimear*, was well used in the twentieth century, is occasionally spelt *Emir*, and has the Scottish Gaelic forms *Eamhair* and *Éimhear*.

## Emmet *m.*

When this surname (which comes from the girl's name Emma) is used as a first name in Ireland it is usually in memory of the United Irishman and patriot Robert Emmet (1778–1803), executed after leading a brief rising against the British in Dublin.

## Ena *f.*

Ena is an anglicized form of both **Eithne** and **Enat**.

Popular in Ireland and Britain in the earlier twentieth century, it is not much used for babies now.

## Enan *Énán* m.

There are said to be nine saints of this name, but its meaning and history are obscure. It is sometimes found as *Éanán*.

## Enat *Aodhnait* f.

Enat is a feminine version of the name **Aidan**, 'little fire'. **Ena**, *Eny* and more rarely *Idnat* are alternative spellings, and many Irish uses of *Enid* (otherwise a Welsh name meaning 'life, soul') belong in this group. There is another unusual Irish name, *Iodhnait* or *Íonait*, meaning 'faithful, sincere', which can also be anglicized as Enat or Enid.

## Enda *Éanna* m.

Enda is traditionally interpreted as meaning 'bird-like' and was the name of an early organiser of Irish monasticism. St Enda (d. c.530) trained in early life as a soldier, and succeeded his father to become ruler of a petty kingdom. According to legend, it was only when he wanted to choose a wife and chose a young woman from the nunnery where his sister St **Fainche** was a nun that, under her guidance, he turned to a religious life. Indeed, in legend Fainche is shown as a major influence in his life. Enda travelled to Scotland to train at St Ninian's famous abbey at Whithorn in Galloway, and returned to Ireland to found several monasteries before settling on Inishmore in the Aran Islands, with which he is particularly associated.

## Eneas *Éneas* m.

This was originally an anglicization of *Éigneachán*, an Irish name and a pet form of *Éigneach*, which probably comes from *écen*, 'force'. It has been re-adapted into Irish as *Éneas*. Éigneachán was also anglicized as *Ignatius*, *Aeneas* and *Neas*, while Eneas was also used as an anglicization of **Aengus**.

## Enid *see* Enat

## Enos *see* Aengus

## Eny *see* Enat

## Enya *see* Eithne

## Eoan *see* Eoghan

## Eochaidh m.

Eochaidh or *Eochaí* means 'horse-rider' and so is probably related to **Eachann**. *Eocho* is its pet form. It was quite common in early times, but the problems of its pronunciation for non-Irish speakers have led to a decline in its use. Attempts to anglicize it have included *Ataigh* and *Atty*, *Eoi*, *Oghe*, *Oghie* and *Oho*. In fiction, two brothers, Eochaidh Feidhleach and Eochaidh Aireamh, were kings of Ireland consecutively in the time of Julius Caesar. As their second names mean 'one who yokes' and 'ploughman', they may refer to some agricultural god. In real life, Eochaidh Éigeas ('the sage or poet') was a prominent sixth-century poet, described in later texts as 'the chief-poet of Ireland'.

### Eoghan *m.*

Eoghan or *Eoan* is taken to mean 'well-born' and is traditionally translated *Eugene* or *Gene*, a Greek name also meaning 'well-born'. The interpretation 'born of the yew' has also been suggested. Eoghan Mór ('the great') founded the Eoghanacht ('race of Eoghan'), the line of early kings of Munster. It has been used steadily since. Eoghan Rua ('the Red') O'Neill (?1590–1649) was a brilliant Irish military leader who in 1646 won a great victory over the Scots Covenanter forces at Benburb. Very different from this aristocrat was the poor bohemian poet Eoghan Rua O Súilleabháin (1748–84), who spent part of his life in the British Navy, press-ganged or fleeing from the womanising for which he was notorious. He was reputed to speak seven languages, had an outstanding gift for poetry and was much admired for his ready wit and outrageous lifestyle. Because of the similarity of sound, the name was often anglicized as *Owen* (the Welsh form of Eugene), as well as *Oyne* or *Oynie*, while in Scotland it was anglicized as *Ewan*, *Ewen*, *Euan* or *Evan*. It is often confused with **Eoin**.

## Eoi *see* Eochaidh

## Eoin *m.*

Eoin is one of the Irish forms of *John*. It was taken directly into Irish from the Latin Iohannes in the early Christian period, while the alternative Irish form **Sean** came into use via the name's French version, Jean. Because the pronunciation of Eoin and **Eoghan** are the same, Eoin has also been anglicized as *Owen* at times; indeed, many people would not distinguish between the two names.

## Erevan *see* Éibhear

## Erin *f.*

*Éire* was the name of an Irish goddess, a sister to **Banba** and **Fódla**. When the Milesians (see **Éibhear**) landed in Ireland, the three goddesses greeted them, each hoping the Milesians would name the country after them. Éire was the winner, although Banba's and Fódla's names are used as poetic terms for Ireland. The island became Éire, and from its form in Irish when it means 'of Éire', comes Erin. The name has been very popular for a number of years in Australia, Canada and the USA, but only recently in Ireland, although Éire was used as an Irish first name in early times. Variant forms have developed, such as *Erinn*, *Eryn*, *Erina* and *Aryn*. One outstanding bearer is the novelist and women's-refuge founder, Erin Pizzey.

### Ernan Earnán m.

This name probably comes from the word *iarn*, 'iron' and was the name of the patron saint of Tory Island. The name *Ernin* (*Eirnín*), which comes from the same word and can be used for either sex, belongs to some eleven saints, including St Ernin Cass ('the curly-haired') of Leighlin.

### Erskine m.

A Scottish surname derived from the place-name. Its meaning is uncertain, although the suggested 'green mantle', indicating a grassy slope. It is found as a first name in Scotland and England as well as in Ireland, where it is associated with (Robert) Erskine Childers (1870-1922), the Republican politician executed during the Civil

War, and author of the still-popular spy novel, *The Riddle of the Sands*.

## Eryn *see* Erin

## Etain *Éadaoin* f.

Etain was one of the Tuatha Dé Danann (see **Dana**), and the most beautiful woman in Ireland. The god Midhir fell in love with her, and won her with the help of **Aengus** Óg, the love god. But Midhir's jealous wife turned her into a fly and called up a wind to blow her far over the ocean. When the fly finally managed to return to Ireland it fell into a cup and was drunk by the wife of one of the warriors of Ulster, who became pregnant. In this way Etain was reborn. Midhir still loved her and tried to win her again, but it was only after many more trials that the lovers were able to escape together in the form of two swans. This story was turned into an opera, *The Immortal Hour*, by Rutland Boughton. First performed in 1914, its huge success led to a brief vogue for the name in both Ireland and England.

## Ethenia, Ethna, Ethni, Etna, Etney *see* Eithne

## Euan, Eugene *see* Eoghan

**Eunan** *see* **Adamnan**

**Eva** *see* **Aoife**

**Evaline** *see* **Evelyn**

**Evan** *see* **Eoghan, Evin**

**Evelyn** *f.*
Evelyn is yet another form of the Irish *Eibhlín* or
*Aibhílín* (see **Aileen** and **Eileen**). Many books on
first names give only *Evelina* and *Eveleen* as Irish
forms of the name, probably because Evelyn is
also used outside Ireland, but while these two
forms, and especially Eveleen, are particularly
Irish, there is no doubt that the form Evelyn is
more common in Ireland than elsewhere. The
name also occurs as *Evaline* and *Evelena*. Evelyn
can, of course, also be used as a masculine name,
as in the novelist Evelyn Waugh, in which case it
comes from the surname, which itself in turn
derives from the first name. However, Evelyn
became so strongly associated with a female
image that the male use is virtually obsolete. The
similar-sounding old Irish name *Evlin* (*Éibhleann*),
means 'sheen, radiance', and may originally have
been the name of a sun-goddess.

### Eveny *Aibhne* m.

This is a name from the Derry area, of obscure meaning and origin. It does not appear until the later Middle Ages, and so does not seem to have belonged to any outstanding character in myth or legend. It is also anglicized as *Aveny*.

### Ever *see* Éibhear

### Evin *Éimhín* m.

From the Irish word *eimh*, 'swift, ready', this name is particularly associated with St Evin, a bishop who gave his name to the monastery he founded at Monasterevan. It is also anglicized as *Evan*.

### Evlin *see* Evelyn

### Ewan, Ewen *see* Eoghan

# f

## Fachnan *Fachtna* m. and f.

This name, more usually male than female, means 'malicious, hostile'. St Fachtna, also known as St *Fachanan* (d. c.600), founded a monastery at Rosscarbery which became the principle centre of learning in west Cork. *Faughnan* is a variant form, and the name was translated *Festus* (as was **Fechin**), even becoming Fantasius in Latin.

## Fainche *f.*

There are fourteen saints of this name, the most famous being the sister of St **Enda**, also known as St *Fanchea*. She was a nun at Rossory on Lough Erne, and according to tradition played a major role as guide and adviser to her more famous brother. The name is also found as *Faenche*.

## Fainne *f.*

*Fainne* is the Irish word for 'ring'. For Irish

speakers it has extra significance as the name of
the lapel badge worn to show they are active Irish-
language users. *Fania* may be an anglicization.

## Fallon *m. and f.*
An Irish surname from Fallamhan or 'leader',
originally a nickname. It came to prominence in
the 1980s through a character in the TV series
*Dynasty*. Not widely adopted, it is still used
occasionally.

## Fanchea *see* Fainche

## Fand *see* Emer

## Fania *see* Fainne

## Faolán *see* Felan

## Farall *see* Farrell

## Fardoragh *Feardorcha m.*
This name means 'dark man', which led to its
literal translation into Latin as Obscurus. In
Donegal it was shortened to *Dorrie*, and it has
also been anglicized as *Firdorcha*. It is translated
*Frederick*.

### Farquhar *Fearchar* m.

The surname Farquhar comes from the early Irish name *Fearchar*, a name meaning 'dear man' or 'friendly'. Although Farquhar is found in Ireland, its use both as a first and surname is primarily associated with the Scottish Highlands.

### Farrell m.

Farrell or *Farall* is an anglicized form of **Fergal**. It was used as a first name in Ireland into the nineteenth century. It also became a common surname, and the name's occasional use in the USA today probably comes directly from the surname.

### Farry *Fearadhach* m.

This name, meaning 'manly', was quite common in early literature, mostly among peripheral characters, although it is also the name of kings in both Ireland and Scotland. In Latin documents the name sometimes misleadingly appears as Fergus.

### Faughnan *see* Fachnan

### Feach, Feagh *see* Fiach

### Fearadhach *see* Farry

**Fearchar** *see* **Farquhar**

**Feardorcha** *see* **Fardoragh**

**Feargal, Fearghal** *see* **Fergal**

**Fearghus** *see* **Fergus**

**Feary** *see* **Fiacre**

**Fechin** *Feichín* m.
This name, which could mean 'raven' or 'battle', belonged to five Irish saints, the most famous of them Fechin of Fore. He was an abbot who founded at least six monasteries and may have visited Scotland, although his name alone may have been taken there by his followers. In either case, it appears there as *Vigean* (sometimes corrupted to Virgin), and he was popular enough for the Scots to develop a first name, Máel Fhéchín, 'servant or devotee of Fechin'. At the parish of St Vigean near Arbroath an annual fair used to be held on St Fechin's feast day, 20 January. He is described in his *Life* as 'a man of a bright, summery life'. Fechin is also anglicized as *Fehin* and translated *Festus*.

**Fedelma** *see* **Fidelma**

### Feenat *Fianait* f.

This name, meaning 'little deer or wild creature', is also found in the forms *Fiadhnait* and *Feena*.

### Fehin, Feichín *see* Fechin

### Feidhelm *see* Fidelma

### Feidhlim, Feidhlimidh *see* Phelim

### Felan *Faolán* m.

This is a common name in early writing, in myth, in religious and in secular life. One holder was a follower of **Finn** Mac Cool, and said to be so loyal that he would rescue Finn from heaven itself; another was a missionary saint who was martyred in Belgium about 656. The name comes from the word for 'wolf' and can also be found as *Phelan*.

### Felim, Felimid, Felimy *see* Phelim

### Fenella *see* Finola

### Feoras m.

An Irish form of *Peter*, via the Norman form Piers (in modern French, Pierre). (See also **Pierce**.)

### Fergal *Fearghal* m.

This popular name means 'valorous'. Fergal Mac Maoldúin was high king of Ireland from 710 to

722. St Fergal, who died in 784, was a missionary monk who preached to the Slavs of Carinthia and became bishop of Salzburg. He is often known as St *Virgil* or *Vergil*, and is one of the few early Irish saints to have been formally canonized. The name also appears as *Feargal* and *Ferghil* and is the source of the name **Farrell**.

## Fergus *Fearghus* m.

Fergus, made up of elements meaning 'man' and 'strength' or 'vigour', was well used in early times and is still popular today. It is used in Scotland and Ireland, for the name forms a link between the two countries. According to tradition, Fergus Mac Erc, Prince of Dál Riada (then north-east Ireland), and his two brothers crossed the seas with his Scots and founded the kingdom of Argyll ('the eastern Gael') in Scotland. This group of Scots (the name of their tribe) became so influential that the whole country was later named after them. Another Fergus linking the two countries is St Fergus, nicknamed 'the Pict', an eighth-century Irish bishop who was a missionary to Scotland.

## Festus *see* Fachnan, Fechin

## Fiach *Fiacha* m.

This name either means 'little raven', or was a pet

form of *Fiachra* (see **Fiacre**). Its most prominent holder was *Feagh* MacHugh O'Byrne (c.1544–97) of Wicklow, who spent a long career harrying the English and their supporters, and won a victory at Glenmalure in 1580. Even after his execution peace was not restored, as his work was continued by his sons **Turlough** and **Phelim**. His name is also anglicized as *Fiach* and *Fiagh*, while in Irish his name is Fiacha or Fiach Mac Aodha Ó Broin.

## Fiacre *Fiachra* m.

Fiacre probably means 'raven'. St Fiacre of Meaux (also known as Fiacre of Breuil) was a hermit who left Ireland as an act of denial and settled in Normandy. There he grew food with such skill that he became the patron saint of horticulture. It has been said that the fact he is also invoked by sufferers from sexually transmitted diseases may be connected with his renowned dislike of women. After his death his relics were taken to Meaux. He was very popular in France, and the Hôtel Saint-Fiacre in Paris was named after him. Cabs operating from outside the hotel came to be called *fiacres*, a name later given to taxis in general, which is how an Irish saint's name entered the international vocabulary and why he is also invoked by travellers. The name has been anglicized as *Feary*.

**Fiadhnait** *see* **Feenat**

**Fiagh** *see* **Feagh**

**Fianait** *see* **Feenat**

## Fidelma *Feidhelm f.*

Fidelma is a name that occurs frequently in early literature: a sorceress of the name was foster-mother to the fifth-century King Conall Corc of Munster; while Fidelma Noíchrothach, ('the nine-times beautiful') was a member of the female champions. As women in early Ireland had, theoretically, equal rights with men in law (hence their prominent role in many stories), some of them, such as the female champions, also fought alongside the men, a Celtic tradition noted as far back as Roman times. The name is also spelt *Fideilme*, and *Fedelma* and is shortened to *Delma*.

## Fina *Fíona f.*

The old Irish name Fíne, from the Latin *vinea,* 'vine', has become Fíona in modern Irish and is anglicized as Fina. The form *Fiona* is also well used in modern Ireland. Users probably do not distinguish between the Irish form and the Scots name Fiona, although language experts do. The Scottish Fiona is an eighteenth-century creation, coined by the poet James Macpherson, apparently as a feminine form of **Finn**, 'white, fair'. It became better-known from Fiona Macleod, the pen-name of Scots writer William Sharp (1855–1905), who specialized as Fiona in Celtic tales and peasant romances, while writing more literary material under his real name. Fiona has become a very popular name in modern Ireland, although it is surprisingly rare in the USA.

## Finan *Fíonán* m.

There are at least nine saints called Finan, including St Finan Cam (d. c.600), founder of the abbey at Kinnity, Co. Offaly; Finan Lobur ('the leper'; in modern Irish *Lobhar*), another sixth-century saint, who was abbot at Swords, north of Dublin; Finan of Aberdeen, also sixth century, preacher to the Scots and the Welsh; and the seventh-century Finan of Lindisfarne, who succeeded **Aidan** and converted the English of Mercia and Essex. The name is also found as *Fionnán* and *Fionan*.

## Finbarr *Fionnbhar* m.

Finbarr or *Fin(n)barr* means 'fair top or hair'. St Finbarr is the patron saint of Cork, about whom miraculous tales are told, such as his riding on horseback over the sea. In folklore, Finbarr was king of the fairies and leader of the fairy host. Well used in Ireland today, the name is also found as *Fionbarra*, *Fionnbhárr* and *Findbarr*, and shortened to **Barry** (a name deriving from Finbarr) and *Barra*.

## Fineen *Fínín* m.

Fineen, which means 'wine-birth', was relatively common in early Ireland. Fineen Fáithliaigh was physician to Conchobhar Mac Nessa (see **Conor**), and in one text appears as a fairy who arrives in a cloud to heal **Cúchulainn**'s wounds; Fineen Mac Luchta was visited every year by a fairy woman who foretold the future; and Fineen Mac Aodha, a real-life king of Munster (d. 619), supposedly became involved with a mythical woman, Mór Mumhan ('Mor of Munster'), who probably represented kingship and the land. It is also found as *Fíngin*, *Finghin*, *Fingin*, *Finneen* and *Finnin*, and was early on translated **Florence**. As a result Florence, as a boy's name, and its short forms *Florry*, *Florrie*, *Flur* and *Flurry*, are still found in Ireland.

## Finella *see* Finola

## Fingal *see* Dougal, Finn

## Finghin, Fingin, Fíngin *see* Fineen

**Finian** see **Finnian**

**Fínín** see **Fineen**

**Finn** *Fionn* m.
Finn means 'white, fair' and the name is closely associated with the hero Finn Mac Cool (Fionn Mac Cuuhaill). His popularity is enduring, for stories about him have been written for over a thousand years. He is still an important figure in Irish literature, appearing in James Joyce's *Finnegans Wake* and **Flann** O'Brien's *At Swim-Two-Birds*. In literary texts Finn is a mighty warrior, leader of the Fianna, the young trainee warriors that form the king's bodyguard. He is wise, brave, good-looking, generous and famed for his cunning in outwitting his enemies. He is sometimes portrayed as a giant. The related name *Fingal* ('fair stranger'; see also **Dougal**), in use in Scotland since the Middle Ages, originally to describe fair-haired Vikings, was used by James Macpherson in his *Ossian* poems for the hero that takes the part of Finn. The name is occasionally found in the form *Fynn*.

**Finnbarr** see **Finbarr**

**Finneen** see **Fineen**

## Finnian *Finnén* m.

Finnian or *Finian* – both are equally well used –
is an interesting name historically, for while the
first part seems to come from the Irish word for
'fair, light', the second half is from the British
rather than Irish form of Celtic. One historian
has even claimed that Finnian is a British form
of **Finbarr**, and that the two famous sixth-century
saints Finnian and Finbarr are the same person.
The former, the abbot of Clonard, Co. Meath, did
indeed have strong British connections, having
studied in Wales and practising a Welsh form of
monasticism at Clonard. He is said to have
attracted three thousand disciples during his
working life, and each monk was sent out with a
gospel book, a crosier and a reliquary to form the
core of a new foundation, whether a monastery
or church. The name's other famous bearer, St
Finnian of Movill, Co. Down, studied in Scotland
rather than Wales. He too was a famous teacher
and scholar who is said to have had St **Columba**
(see **Colm**) among his students. In the twentieth-
century the name Finnian has been given world-
wide publicity by the stage musical and film,
*Finian's Rainbow* (1968).

## Finnin *see* Fineen

## Finola *Fionnuala* f.

This name, popular in the twentieth century, means 'fair or white shoulder' and is used equally in its anglicized and native Irish forms. Finola MacDonnell was the mother of the famous Red Hugh O'Donnell (?1571–1602). The daughter of a Scottish Highland chief, she was described by a contemporary as one who 'joined a man's heart to a woman's thought', and was to a large extent the driving force behind her son's rising. She was known affectionately as Ineen Duv ('the Dark Lady'; Iníon Dubh in modern Irish), and some sources treat this, in the form *Ineenduv*, as her first name. Another Highland woman of virtually the same name was Flora Macdonald (1722–90), famous for helping Bonnie Prince Charlie during his flight after the Battle of Culloden (1746). She was really a Finola, or the Scottish form *Fenella*, Flora being a standard translation of the name. There is an alternative, little-used Irish spelling of the name, *Fionnghuala*. It is also anglicized as *Finella*, and its short form, **Nuala**, is now so well used as to count as an independent name.

## Fintan *Fiontan* m.

Fintan is another name from the Irish word for 'white, fair'. There are some seventy-four Irish saints of this name, including the best known, St Fintan of Clonenagh (d. 603), a man who was strict with himself – he was said to have lived on a diet of barley bread and clayey water – but whose many acts of kindness to others are recorded; St Fintan of Munnu (d. 635), rejected as a monk by St **Columba**'s abbey at Iona on the grounds that he should instead be an abbot himself; and St Fintan of Rheinau (d. 879) who was captured by Vikings, taken as a slave to Orkney, escaped, made his way to Rome and ended his life as a hermit on an island in the Rhine. His relics are still at Rheinau. A more recent holder of the name was James Fintan Lalor (1807–49), a land agitator and member of the Young Ireland group. The name is also found as *Fionntán*.

**Fiona, Fíona** see **Fina**

**Fionan, Fíonán, Fionnán** see **Finan**

**Fionn** see **Finn**

**Fionnbhar, Fionnbhárr, Fionbharra** see **Finbarr**

**Fionnghuala** see **Finola**

**Fionntán** see **Fintan**

**Fionnuala** *see* **Finola**

**Fiontan** *see* **Fintan**

**Firdorcha** *see* **Fardoragh**

### Fírinne *f.*

From the Irish word for 'truth', this name could be seen as a literal translation of the name *Verity*.

### Fítheal, Flaithrí *see* **Florence**

### Flann *m. and f.*

Flann means 'bright blood red'. It was a popular name in the past, and one royal Flann of the tenth century left a great stone cross at Clonmacnoise, carved with scenes from the scriptures. The best-known modern user is probably the author **Brian** O'Nolan (1911–66) who used Flann O'Brien as one of his pen-names. In the past Flann was also a girl's name, but is less likely to be so today.

### Flannan *Flannán m.*

Flannan is a pet form of **Flann**, and the name of a seventh-century saint and bishop venerated in both Ireland and Scotland. While the remains of his stone oratory can still seen beside the cathedral of Killaloe, Co. Clare, he was also a wandering preacher. The Flannan Islands in the Hebrides, to the west of Lewis and Harris, are named after the ruined chapel dedicated to him on one of the islands, all that remains of an early monastery.

## Flannchadh *see* Clancy

## Flannery *m. and f.*
This Irish surname, which comes from an old name meaning '(with) red eyebrows', is occasionally used as a first name. Its use as a female first name is shown in the writer Flannery O'Connor.

## Flora, Florence *see* Bláthnait

## Florence *m.*
In the Middle Ages Florence was a Europe-wide male name, taken from the Latin word for 'blooming'. Its use as a girl's name dates only from the fame of Florence Nightingale, so-called because she was born in the Italian city. Florence survived in Ireland as a boy's name long after it fell from favour elsewhere because it was used to translate a number of Irish names including **Fineen**, *Fítheal* ('goblin'), and **Flann**. *Florry*, *Florrie*, *Flur* or *Flurry* were also used as pet forms of these names, and Florry or Flurry is still quite common today as the anglicization of *Flaithrí*, 'lord and king'.

**Flur, Flurry** *see* **Fineen, Florence**

**Flynn** *m. and f.*

This Irish surname, a version of **Flann**, 'bright blood red', has recently come into use as a first name for both sexes. No doubt its appeal is helped by the glamour attached to the Australian actor Errol Flynn, himself of Irish background.

**Frances, Francis, Frank(ie)** *see* **Proinsias**

**Fynn** *see* **Finn**

# g

**Gabriel** *see* **Gay**

**Gael** *m.*
In mythology, Gael is the name given to the man from whom all the Gaelic peoples are descended. This is a typical ancestor tale of the sort invented to explain the name of different groups of people.

**Galway** *m.*
This unusual man's name, occasionally used in the USA, as with the poet Galway Kinnell, comes from the Irish place-name. The name of Galway town, and hence the county, comes from the Irish *gall*, 'stone', and so means 'stony'. But *gall* is also Irish for 'stranger, foreigner' (used first to describe the Vikings, then the English), and the name is sometimes popularly understood to be from this.

**Garbhán** *see* **Garvin**

## Garret *Gearóid* m.

An Irish form of the name **Gerald** introduced into Ireland by its Norman conquerors, this name came into use either directly or by way of the surname (which can also come from **Gerard**). The former Taioseach (Prime Minister) Garret Fitzgerald represents one spelling of the name, and actor *Garrett* Keogh another. A very popular name in Ireland, it is used as an Irish translation of both Gerald and Gerard. It has become fairly popular in the USA recently, also occurring as *Gerrit*, while *Gary* or *Garry* is sometimes considered a short form.

## Garvin *Garbhán* m.

This name comes from the word for 'rough'. *Garvan* is an alternative spelling.

## Garry *see* Garret

## Gay m.

While in other countries Gay is a dying feminine name, in Ireland, and especially in Dublin, this is a standard form of the boy's name *Gabriel*, a biblical name meaning 'man of God'. Gay Byrne is a famous TV and radio presenter.

## Gearalt *see* Gerald

## Gearárd *see* Gerard

**Gearóid** *see* **Garret**

**Gearóidín** *see* **Geraldine**

**Gene** *see* **Eoghan**

**Geoffrey** *see* **Séafraid, Seathrún, Siothrún**

**George** *see* **Seoirse**

**Ger** *m.*
An Irish short form of both **Gerald** and **Gerard**.

## Gerald *Gearalt* m.

This name comes from Germanic words meaning 'spear' and 'rule'. In 1097 the Norman Gerald of Windsor was put in charge of Pembroke Castle in Wales. It was his sons and grandsons, known as the FitzGeralds ('sons or descendants of Gerald') or the Geraldines, who some sixty years later came to Ireland at the invitation of **Dermot**, King of Leinster. Better equipped and better disciplined that the Irish, these Normans ended the Irish royal line and started over eight hundred years of rule from England. The Anglo–Saxon form of the name was recorded in Ireland before then, as in St Gerald of Mayo (d. 732), an Englishman who was a monk at Lindisfarne before moving to Ireland; but it was the Fitzgeralds who really introduced it to Ireland. It is still very common today, whether in its full form or shortened to *Gerry* and **Ger**.

## Geraldine *Gearóidín f.*

One of the descendants of the Norman **Gerald** was a sixteenth-century Lady Elizabeth Fitzgerald. The English courtier-poet the Earl of Surrey wrote a poem praising the beauty of the 'fair Geraldine'. This was the origin of the name, although it did not become popular until the nineteenth century. It has been well used in Ireland since then, and is found throughout the English-speaking world.

## Gerard *Gearárd m.*

This name, from Germanic words meaning 'spear' and 'brave', was introduced by the Normans along with **Gerald**. Not surprisingly the two names were often confused, and Gerard was rather swamped by Gerald. However, it is common in Ireland today, probably because of the popularity of St Gerard Majella (d. 1755. See also **Majella**). *Giorárd* is an alternative Irish form of the name, and it can be shortened to *Gerry* or **Ger**.

## Gerrit *see* **Garret**

**Gerry** *see* **Gerald, Gerard**

## 'Gil-' prefixed names *see* **Gillespie**

## Gillespie *Giolla Easpie* m.

Many Irish and Scottish surnames begin with
'Gil-' or 'Gill-', and these come from a common
name element in early names – *giolla*, 'servant' or
'devotee', which was then followed by the name
of a saint or object of service. Some of these have
survived through the ages as first names, and
some have been re-adopted from surnames.
Gillespie means 'servant of the bishop', *Gilpatrick*
(*Giolla Pádraig*) was a devotee of St **Patrick**,
*Gilbride* (*Giolla Bhríde*) devotee of St **Brigid**,
*Gilchrist* (*Giolla Chríst*, sometimes translated
'Christian') a servant of Christ, and so on.

## Giorárd *see* **Gerard**

## Gobnet *Gobnait* f.

This name, traditionally interpreted as coming
from *gob*, 'mouth', belonged to a fifth-century saint
who gave her name to Kilgobnet, Co. Kerry, where
she founded a church. She was a skilled bee-
keeper, and a number of miracles are attributed to
her. The name is still in use and has several
anglicized forms, including *Gobnat*, *Gobinet*,

*Gubby* and *Webby*. It was translated as *Barbara* (see **Baibin**).

## Gofraidh *see* Corey

## Gormlaith *f.*

Gormlaith means 'illustrious lady', and was the name of one of the most extraordinary women in Irish history, who sometimes appears in the history books as *Gormflath*. She was a princess of the royal line of Leinster, sister to the king, and managed to be both the wife of **Brian** Boru, the great enemy of the Vikings in Ireland, and the mother of **Sitric** Silk-beard, Viking king of Dublin. Gormlaith had first been married to Olaf, leader of the Dublin Vikings, by whom she had Sitric. She then married **Malachy**, High King of Ireland, and when rejected by him, married Brian. One modern historian has said she was 'one of the fateful women of Irish history. Her career was long and disastrous for Ireland, however much she justified it as a Leinster patriot and for the sake of husband and brother'; while a Norse saga, where her name becomes 'Kormlada', says she was 'fairest and best-gifted in everything that was not in her own power, but it was the talk of men that she did all things ill over which she had any power'. *Gormla* is a modern Irish spelling of her name, which can take the form *Gormelia* in Scotland.

## Grania *Gráinne f.*

Grania is a name which either comes from a word meaning 'grain, corn' or else means 'she who inspires terror'. It is the name of the heroine of one of the great Irish love-stories, which is told under the name of her lover, **Dermot**. The name was translated Grace, which is why the pirate Gráinne Ní Mháille is usually to be found in the history books as Grace O'Malley (?1530–?1600). She led the sea-faring O'Malleys in her own right, raiding successfully even as far as Scotland, as well as gaining power through her marriages. Stories of her bravery are still current in Connacht folklore. She also sailed to London to submit to Elizabeth I and, according to the story, these two formidable women, communicating in Latin, liked one another. Her name passed into poetry as a symbol of Ireland. The commonest anglicized form is the phonetic *Grania*, but others include *Grainne*, *Granya*, *Granna* and *Granina*.

## Gubby *see* Gobnet

# h

**Hamish** *see* **Seamus**

**Hanorah** *see* **Honor**

**Heber, Heremon, Hermon** *see* **Éibhear**

**Hector** *see* **Eachann**

**Hewney** *see* **Owny**

**Hierlath** *see* **Jarlath**

**Honor** *Onóra f.*
An Irish form of the name *Honora* from the Latin
Honoria, 'honour' Another form is *Hanorah*, while
its short forms are the source of **Nora** and **Noreen**.

**Hugh** *see* **Aodh**

**Humphrey** *see* **Auliffe**

# Í

**Iagan** *see* **Egan**

**Iarfhlaith, Iarlaith** *see* **Jarlath**

**Ibar** *see* **Ivar**

**Ida, Íde** *see* **Ita**

**Idnat** *see* **Enat**

**Ignatius** *see* **Eneas**

**Ilene** *see* **Eileen**

**Ina** *Aghna f.*
In Ireland Ina probably represents an Irish form of
the name *Agnes* (otherwise *Aignéis*) but elsewhere
it is usually a short form of any name ending '-ina'.

**Ineenduv** *see* **Finola**

**Iobhar** *see* **Ivar**

**Iodhnait, Íonait** *see* **Enat**

**Iósep, Ióseph** *see* **Seosamh**

**Irial** *m.*

This name of unknown meaning is found in early records and has been revived in recent years.

**Isabel** *see* **Sibéal**

**Iseult** *f.*

The origin of this name is obscure, although it is certainly Celtic. Esyllt, the Welsh form of the name, has been interpreted as meaning 'of fair aspect'. In Arthurian romance Iseult was an Irish princess, skilled in medicine. She was destined to marry old King Mark of Cornwall, and his dashing nephew Tristan came to bring her from Ireland. By mistake they drank the love-potion Iseult's mother had provided to ensure her marriage with Mark was happy, and the two were condemned to adulterous love for the rest of their lives. The name was chosen by the Irish patriot Maud Gonne for her daughter, and can appear as *Isolda*, *Isolde*, *Yseult* and in other variations.

**Isleen** *see* **Aislinn**

**Isobel** *see* **Sibéal**

**Isolda, Isolde** *see* **Iseult**

### Ita *Íde f.*

A fairly common girl's name, Ita probably comes from the old Irish word for 'thirst'. It was borne by Ireland's most famous woman saint after **Brigid**. Known as 'the foster-mother of the saints' after the number she educated, her wise advice was much in demand. She also wrote an Irish lullaby to the Infant Jesus. Ita is anglicized as *Ida*, although this can also be a Germanic name meaning 'work'.

### Ivar *Iobhar m.*

Ivar is another Irish masculine name which comes from a tree name. As **Dara** comes from the oak, Ivar means 'yew'. First names from the name of this important tree can be traced in all Celtic languages. St Ibar or *Ibar* of Begerin (Wexford harbour) so inspired one early writer that he likened him to 'a splendid flame over a sparkling wave'.

# j

### Jacinta *f.*
This is a Spanish name, a form of the name Hyacinth, that is also used in Ireland. Examples of holders are the artist Jacinta Feeney and the opera singer Jacinta Malcahy.

### Jane *see* **Síne, Sinead, Siobhan**

### Jarlath *Iarlaith* m.
St Jarlath (d. c.550) is the patron saint of Tuam, Co. Galway, and the name is still particularly to be found in that area. St Jarlath, bishop of Tuam, was said to have been from a local noble family. The monastery he established became a centre of learning. The name is also found as *Hierlath* and *Iarfhlaith*.

### Jerome, Jeremiah *m.*
These otherwise unfashionable names are found

in Ireland because they were traditionally used to translate the name **Dermot**. *Jarmy* is another form the name took.

## Joan *see* **Sinead, Siobhan, Siún**

## John *see* **Eoin, Sean, Seón, Shane**

## Joseph *see* **Seosamh**

## Josephine *see* **Seosaimhín**

## Junan, Junanan *see* **Adamnan**

## Juno *f.*
Juno, the name of the Roman queen of the gods, was used to translate **Una**. The name was brought to prominence by **Sean** O'Casey's play, *Juno and the Paycock* (1924), but evidence for its real-life use is hard to find.

## Juverna *f.*
This is another term for Ireland – this time a Latin one – which is occasionally used as a first name.

# k

**Kacey** *m. and f.*
This, along with *Kacee*, *Kacie*, *Kaci* and *Kasey*, are American spellings of **Casey**.

**Kaelan** *see* **Keelin**

**Kaine** *see* **Kane**

**Kaitlyn** *f.*
This spelling of **Caitlin** has become very popular in the USA, reflecting the way it is pronounced there, as if a blend of Kate and Lyn. It is also found as *Kaitlin*, *Kaitlynn*, *Katelyn(n)*, *Katelin* and *Kaytlin*. It is now well used in Ireland.

**Kálmán** *see* **Colman**

**Kane** *Cathán m.*
Kane is the anglicization of the old Irish name Cathán, from *cath*, or 'battle', so the name would

mean something like 'warrior'. It appears as
Chattan in the person of St Chattan of Kingarth,
a sixth-century Irishman who travelled to Scotland
where he founded several churches around the
Clyde before moving to the Isle of Bute to found
the monastery of Kingarth. Kane has been well
used in Australia and is also used in the USA,
where it is can be found as *Kaine* and *Kayne*.

**Kary** *see* **Carey**

**Kasey** *see* **Casey, Kacey**

**Kassidi, Kassidy** *see* **Cassidy**

**Katelin, Katelyn(n)** *see* **Kaitlyn**

**Kathel** *see* **Cahal**

**Kathleen** *f.*
Kathleen is the anglicized form of **Caitlin**, the Irish
form of *Catherine* (see **Catriona**). It featured
regularly in the top ten names of the English-
speaking world in the earlier twentieth century, but
its popularity is now declining except in the USA,
where both it and Caitlin are increasingly popular.
From the eighteenth century the figure of *Kathleen
Ní Houlihan* appears in Irish songs as a symbol of

Ireland, with the fight to make Kathleen a queen once again representing the struggle for an independent Ireland. The name is also spelt *Cathleen*.

### Katrine *Caitrín* f.
This is yet another Irish version of the name *Catherine*. (See **Catriona**, **Caitlin** and **Kathleen**.)

### Kaylyn *see* **Keelin**

### Kayne *see* **Kane**

### Kaytlin *see* **Kaitlyn**

### Keagan *see* **Keegan**

### Kealan *see* **Kelan**

### Kean *Cian* m.
This name means 'ancient'. It was the name of **Brian** Boru's son-in-law, who led the troops from **Desmond** against the Vikings in the Battle of Clontarf in 1014, where both he and his father-in-law were killed. There are several variants of the name, including *Kian*, *Keane* and *Cain*, an unfortunate form because of its association with one of the arch-villains of the Bible. (See also **Kenan**.)

## Keara *see* Ciara

## Keavy *Caoimhe f.*

Keavy or Keeva comes from a word with several meanings, including 'precious', 'beloved', 'beautiful' and 'graceful'. It is related to the boy's name **Kevin**. Caoimhe is currently popular in Ireland.

## Kedagh *Céadach m.*

A well-used name in the later Middle Ages. Its meaning is unclear, but it may come from a word for 'first', or from a word meaning 'hundred'.

## Keegan *m.*

This Irish surname is being well used in the USA as a boy's name. It comes from Mac Aodhagain, meaning 'son of Aeducan', a pet form of **Aodh**, 'fire'. It is also spelt *Keagan* and *Keegen*.

## Keelan *see* Killian

## Keeley, Keelie *see* Keely

## Keelin *Caoilfhionn f.*

This name, of an Irish virgin saint, comes from the words *caol*, 'slender', and *fionn*, 'fair, white, pure'. The Irish form of the name can also be spelt *Caoilinn* or *Caelainn*. *Kaylyn* is a popular girl's name in the USA. While it can be derived from a simple blend of Kay and Lyn, some parents use it as a form of the Irish name, in which case it can also be spelt in ways such as *Caylin* and *Kaelan*.

## Keely *f.*
Used in Ireland and in Britain, this name is also growing in popularity in the USA. It can be thought of as a form of **Keelin** or of Kayleigh, but is probably best interpreted as a feminine form of **Kiely** (also an alternative spelling), from *cadhla*, 'beautiful, graceful'. It is often spelt *Keeley*, and can also be found as *Keelie*, *Keily* and *Keylee*. The dancer Keely Garfield and the singer Keely Smith are American examples of bearers of the name.

**Keenan** *see* **Kenan**

**Keenat** *see* **Kinnat**

**Keenen, Keenon** *see* **Kenan**

**Keera** *see* **Kira**

**Keily** *see* **Keely**

**Keira** *see* **Kira**

## Kelan *Caolán* m.

Meaning 'slender lad', Kelan belongs in the same name-group as **Keelin**. It is also spelt *Kealan*. The various names starting with a 'k' sound and with an 'l' in the middle are always in danger of being confused, and it is probably unwise to insist on distinguishing them too precisely.

## Kelly *Ceallach* m. and f.

This is one of the Irish names that has conquered the world. At the moment it is more often found used for boys in the USA than elsewhere. But as a girl's name it belongs in the lists of most popular names in Britain, Australia and particularly the USA. It seems a pity, therefore that its meaning is not clear. It was traditionally interpreted as 'frequenter of churches' or as deriving from a word for 'strife', but is now thought to mean 'bright-headed'. This confusion does not worry most parents, who use it simply for its strong Irish connections. One bearer was Ceallach Mac Aodh, better known as St *Celsus*, who was archbishop of Armagh from 1105 to 1129. A keen reformer, he was the last hereditary or familial holder of the post. The Irish name is also spelt *Ceallagh*, and a pet form or the name, *Ceallachán*, is the source of the surname and first name **Callaghan**.

### Kenan *Cianán* m.

A pet form of the name *Cian* (see **Kean**), this name is better-known as the surname *Keenan*, which is enjoying a moderate popularity at the moment in the USA as a first name. It is also found as *Keenen*, *Keenon* and *Kienan*.

### Kennan m.

An Irish surname from Mac Fhionnáin, 'son of the fair one', which is sometimes used as a first name.

### Kennedy *f. and m.*

An Irish surname from O Cinnéide, also a surname, or 'son of *Cinnéide*', an Irish first name still in use, meaning 'ugly-headed'. Its use as a first name owes much to respect for the US political family, and especially President John F. Kennedy (1917–63).

### Kenneth m.

This is a name with two sources, one **Canice**, the other **Cináed** or **Cionnaodh**, interpreted as meaning 'born of fire', but quite possibly an Irish borrowing of a Pictish name. It was used by the Irish for Kenneth Mac Alpin, the great ninth-century warrior-king who was the first ruler of both the Picts and Scots, effectively forming the kingdom of Scotland. The name is associated more with Scotland than Ireland, but has been used in Ireland since the eighth century. *Kenny* is used as a short form and also as a direct anglicization of **Canice**.

## Keri *see* **Kerry**

## Kermit *m.*
This name, widely known from *The Muppets* TV series, is in fact a form of the surname MacDermot (son of **Dermot**), *Kermode* being a better-known form of the name. It was borne by a son of American president Theodore Roosevelt.

## Kerry *f. and m.*
Kerry is a place-name used as a first name. At first mainly a masculine name, as in the Australian business magnate Kerry Packer, it is now still used for both sexes, but more often for girls. In the USA Kerry is the usual masculine spelling, but as a girl's name it is more often spelt *Keri*. It also occurs as *Kerri* and *Kerrie*. The Irish form of the place-name is Ciarraí, and it means 'land of the descendants of Ciar'. Ciar is usually a feminine name, meaning 'black' (see **Ciara**), but in the case of Ciarraí it refers to a son of the legendary Queen **Maeve**, whose descendants

were believed to occupy the land. New names such as *Kerryn* could be seen as developments of the name Kerry, or even as a form of the Irish surname Kerrin, which comes from the related name **Kieran**.

## Kevin *Caoimhín* m.

On a global scale, Kevin is probably the most popular Irish masculine name at the moment. It took off in Ireland in the 1920s, was high in the British popularity stakes by 1950 (although it peaked by the end of the 1970s), was one of the top dozen names in the USA in the 1970s and is very popular there again at the moment, and in 1994 was the most popular name for baby boys in France. The name means 'beautiful birth (i.e. child)', and was the name of St Kevin (d. c.618), founder and abbot of the great monastery at Glendalough, one of the most beautiful of the many imposing monastery sites in Ireland. The name is occasionally spelt *Keven*, and *Kevan* is often treated as a variant, although it can also be from the related Irish name *Caomhán*, 'beloved person, friend'.

## Keylee *see* Keely

## Keyra *see* Kira

**Kian** *see* **Kean**

**Kiely** *Cadla* m.
Kiely is related to **Kevin**, coming from the same root meaning 'beautiful, comely'. (See also **Keely**.)

**Kienan** *see* **Kenan**

**Kiera** *see* **Ciara, Kira**

**Kieran** *Ciarán* m.
This is another name which, as well as being popular in Ireland, has been successful elsewhere. The name comes from the word 'dark', which also lies behind the name's modern feminine equivalent, **Ciara**, and the old Irish one, *Ciarnait*. The anglicized Kieran seems to be the commonest form of the name, especially outside Ireland, but the form *Ciaran* is also well used, especially among younger people. It can also be found spelt *Kyran* and *Kieron*. There are twenty-six saints Kieran in Ireland, the earliest probably being St Kieran of Seir, Co. Offaly, said to have been made bishop by St **Patrick**. The most famous bearer is St Kieran of Clonmacnoise (c.512–545; his name is also found in the forms *Ceran* and *Queran*). Of humble origin, he was the son of a travelling

carpenter, while most monastic founders were from noble families. Nevertheless, his foundation became one of the great centres of religion and worship in Ireland, and despite being frequently raided by Vikings and the English, survived as an active monastery until 1552. The Clonmacnoise crosier, now in the National Museum, Dublin, may have been his.

## Killian *Cillian* m.

There are two views about the meaning of Killian. One is that it comes from a word for 'strife', the other that it comes from a word meaning 'church, (monastic) cell'. Of the saints bearing this name, two are connected with the Continent. St Killian of Aubigny was a contemporary of St **Fiacre**, and the same bishop of Meaux, St Faro, found them both hermitages in France. St Killian of Wurzburg is the only Irish saint whose feast is celebrated liturgically in Germany, and his name is used there. Killian and eleven companions travelled to this area of Germany to convert Gozbert, the local duke, and his people. Gozbert became a Christian, but when Killian tried to end the marriage of Gozbert and his brother's widow (they were too closely related for the marriage to be acceptable to the Church),

he was assassinated. The name is often spelt
*Kilian*, and *Keelan* is a variant.

## Kinnat *Ciannait f.*

Kinnat or *Keenat* is a feminine form of *Cian*
(see **Kean**), meaning 'ancient' or 'enduring'.

## Kira *f.*

Kira is an American feminine form of **Kieran**,
no doubt developed because of the complications
of using **Ciara** in the USA (see that entry for
further information). The name is also found as
*Keera*, *Keira*, *Keyra*, *Kiera* and *Kirra*.

## Kodee, Kodi(e), Kody *see* Cody

## Kolman *see* Colman

## Korey, Korri, Korry *see* Corey

## Kyne *Cadhan m.*

Kyne, found occasionally in the USA, is an old
Derry name meaning 'wild goose'. In the local
folklore, Kyne and his magical hound killed a
monster that had been terrorising the area.

## Kyran *see* Kieran

# L

## Labhrás *m.*

Labhrás is the Irish form of *Laurence*, 'man from (the Roman town of) Laurentum'. It is also found as *Labhras* or *Lubhrás*, and the pet form Larry becomes *Learai* in Irish. It was adopted out of respect for St Laurence the Librarian (d. 258), surely the only heroic figure from that misunderstood profession, who was martyred by being roasted on a gridiron after he refused to hand over the Church's money and books. The name was introduced by the Normans. Laurence is also used as a translation of **Lochlann** and **Lorcan**. St Laurence O'Toole is dealt with under Lorcan, his native name.

## Lachann, Lachie, Lachlan, Lachlann *see* Lochlann

## Lachtna *m.*

Lachtna and its pet form *Lachtnán* would have

started as nicknames, for they mean 'milk-like'. Lachtna is one source for the Irish use of **Lucius**.

## Laisren, Laisrián *see* Laserian

## Lana, Lanna *see* Alannah

## Lanty *Leachlainn m.*
This is a shortened form of Maoilseachlann (or Maeleachlainn), 'devotee of St Sechnall or Secundinus', which is anglicized to **Malachy**. The anglicization *Laughlin* is shared with **Lochlann**.

## Laoighseach, Laoiseach *see* Lysagh

## Laoise *f.*
As well as being an Irish place-name, Laoise, probably a form of **Luíseach** (see *Lughaidh*), is an increasingly popular first name. The form *Leesha* shows its pronunciation. Laoise Kelly is a prominent young Irish harpist.

## Lasair, Lasairíona *see* Lassarina

## Laserian *Lasairian, Laisrián m.*
This name means 'little fire'. St Laserian, also known as *Laisren* and *Molaise* or *Molaisse* ('Mo-' in front of a name in Irish signifies 'my', and is a sign of affection), was an Irish monk, possibly a bishop, who had connections with both Ireland

and Scotland but is particularly associated with a healing well at Leighlin, Co. Carlow, where he was abbot. It is said that he voluntarily became ill with thirty illnesses at once, choosing suffering in this life to avoid it in the next. The sick still turn to him and his well. In the north the name has been anglicized to Lazarus, no doubt because the Bible story of the beggar who suffered in this life and thereby merited heaven, recalled Laserian.

## Lassarina *Lasairíona* f.

Lassarina or *Lasrina* means 'fire of wine'. *Lassar* (*Lasair*), meaning 'flame, fire', was a simpler form of the name and common in early times.

## Laughlin *see* Lanty, Lochlann

## Laurence *see* Labhrás, Lochlann, Lorcan

## Leachlainn *see* Lanty

## Leahdan *see* Liadan

## Lean *Léan* f.

An Irish pet form of Eleanore or Eleanora, which become *Eiléanór* or *Eileanóir* and *Eilíonóra* in Irish.

## Leanan *see* Liadan

## Learai *see* Labhrás

**Leesha** *see* **Laoise**

**Lelia** *see* **Lila**

**Lewy** *see* **Lughaidh**

## Liadan *Líadán f.*

Liadan, whose name means 'grey lady', was a
poet and nun from Munster who fell in love with
the poet Cuirithir. As their love was forbidden,
he became a monk and went to live in Waterford.
When he heard that Liadan was coming to visit
him he left, sailing across the sea in his coracle.
Liadan came to the flagstone where Cuirithir used
to pray and stayed on it, sorrowfully, until she died.
She was buried below it. Their story has been
described as the Irish Abelard and Eloise. The
name's Irish form can also be spelt *Líadáin* and
*Líadáine*, and in the USA, where it is occasionally
found, it can be spelt *Liadaine* and *Leahdan*. There
is also a masculine equivalent, *Leanan* (*Liadhnán*).

## Liam *m.*

This enormously popular name is a short form of
**Uilliam**, the Irish form of *William*, but is now so
well established it has all but replaced the fuller
form. William is a Germanic name from elements
meaning 'will, desire' and 'helmet, protection'.

### Life *f.*

Tradition says that this was the name of the woman who gave her name to the River Liffey that flows though Dublin. This is a pleasant story, but unfortunately seems to have been made up to account for the name of the river, which otherwise cannot be explained. (See also **Anna Livia**.)

### Lila *Líle f.*

Lila is an anglicized form of the Irish name *Lil* or *Líle*, which may be a pet form of the name Elizabeth. It is also anglicized as *Lelia* and *Lilly*.

### Lochlann *Lochlainn m.*

Norway was known as the 'land of the lochs', this name's probable origin. A Norwegian would mean a Viking to the people of Ireland and the Scots of the Western Isles. As the Vikings and Irish intermarried, the name lost its sense of 'foreigner'. In Ireland it was anglicized as *Laughlin* (see also **Lanty**) and *Loughlin*, and translated *Laurence*. In the Gaelic of the Scottish Highlands it became *Lachlann* and *Lachann*, and was anglicized as *Lachlan*. This is the form which spread to other countries: emigrating Highlanders took the name to Canada where the Scots pet form *Lachie* became *Lockie*. The name was also taken to Australia, where it has been very popular for the last twenty years. Its spread in Australia was no doubt helped by the fame of General Lachlan Macquarie, governor of New South Wales from 1809 to 1821, after whom Australia's native form of late-Georgian architecture – Macquarie Style – is named.

## Loman *Lomán* m.

This name, from the Irish word for 'bare', was the name of a saint said to be a nephew of St **Patrick**. He became bishop of Trim, Co. Meath, and died about 450. This saint is sometimes called *Lonan* (*Lonán*), but this is a different name which comes from the word for 'blackbird'. Since there are at least four saint Lomans and at least eleven saint Lonans, it is not surprising that a slip of the pen or tongue would cause confusion.

## Lorcan *Lorcán* m.

This name comes from *lorc*, 'silent' or 'fierce', and is translated *Laurence*. The saint known in English as Laurence O'Toole (?1130–80) is in Irish Lorcán Ó Tuathail. As bishop of Dublin at the time of the Norman invasion he was involved in affairs of state, acting as a mediator between the invaders and the Irish, and as an emissary to the English

King Henry II. He was also a church reformer, visited Rome and became a papal legate, and was outstanding in his relief of the poor of his diocese.

### Loretta, Loretto *f.*

Loreto in Italy became a centre of pilgrimage when the holy house of the Virgin Mary was allegedly transported there from Nazareth by angels in the thirteenth century. The place-name was used as a girl's first name by devout parents, and is usually found in the form Loretta, which avoids the problem of the '-o' ending's being masculine in Italian. It is used by Catholics throughout the world, but particularly in Ireland.

### Loughlin *see* Lochlann

### Louis *see* Aloysius, Lughaidh

### Lubhrás *see* Labhrás

### Lucius *m.*

Lucius is an ancient Roman name from the word for 'light'. It was well used in Ireland into the nineteenth century as a translation of **Lachtna** and *Laoighseach* (see **Lysagh**). In the past it was so strongly identified with the Irish that the Irish dramatist Richard Brinsley Sheridan used the name for a stereotypical, hot-headed, comic Irishman in his play *The Rivals* (1775).

## Lughaidh *m.*
Lugh of the Long Arm was an early Irish god, described as 'master of all the arts', whose name means 'light, brightness' or 'the shining one'. This links him with early sun gods, and forms of his name are to be found throughout the Celtic areas. Lughaidh comes from this god's name, and was a very popular name in early times. It can also be spelt *Lúí* and was anglicized by the phonetic spelling *Lewy*. Not surprisingly, this was identified with a short or phonetic form of *Louis* (or Lewis), and this was used to translate it. **Aloysius** is also a form of the name Louis, which explains how Aloysius came to be used as a translation of the apparently unrelated Lughaidh. *Luighseach* or *Luíseach*, 'radiant girl', is a related feminine name.

## Lysagh *Laoiseach m.*
Lysagh, meaning 'man of Laois', was translated **Lucius** or Lewis. It can also be spelt *Laoighseach*.

# m

**Mab, Mabbie, Mabbina** *see* **Maeve**

**Mac Beatha, Macbeth** *see* **Betha**

**Mac Dara** *see* **Dara**

**Macha** *f.*
Macha was the Ulster goddess of sovereignty, although she is often described as a goddess of war. She gave her name to Emain Macha (the great earthworks at Navan Fort near Armagh) which was the royal centre for Ulster, and also to Armagh, 'the height of Macha'. There is also a patroness of Killiney, Co. Kerry, called St Macha.

**Maedóc** *see* **Malachy**

**Maeleachlainn, Máelechlainn** *see* **Malachy**

**Maelisa** *see* **Maoilíosa**

## Maeve *Meadhbh* f.

This name means 'she who intoxicates'. Maeve, like Macha, was an Irish goddess of sovereignty, and so was depicted in story as having several husbands or partners, as every king is in a sense married to her. She was best known for her part in the Táin Bó Cuailnge (the Cattle Raid of Cooley), which she instigated and which led to the death of **Cúchullain**. Here again her role was symbolic, for the story represents the struggles for the high kingship between the Connacht holders and the royal line of Ulster. The name has also been anglicized as *Mave*, *Meave*, *Mab* (Shakespeare's Mab of the Fairies is probably an echo of her name) and *Mabbie*. The Irish form can also be spelt *Meibh*. *Meaveen* or *Mabbina* (*Meidhbhín*) is the pet form. The name was popular from the 1930s to the '50s. The author Maeve Binchy is a well-known bearer.

## Maghnus, Magnus *see* Manus

## Mahon *Mathúin* m.

This is a contracted form of *Mathghamhain*, 'little bear', which was held by the tenth-century King of Cashel, brother of the great **Brian** Boru.

## Maidie *f.*

Seemingly a pet form of 'maiden', this name is, for no known reason, popular in Scotland and Ireland.

## Maighread, Maighréad *see* Mairead

## Maille, Mailse, Mailti *see* Maire

## Mainchín *see* Mannix

## Maire *Máire f.*

Until the sixteenth century the name of Christ's mother was, out of respect, little used in Ireland. It later became very popular and developed many different forms, although Muire is still reserved for the Virgin Mary. Today the simpler forms of *Mary* are out of fashion but many Irish variants are well used (see **Maura**, **Maureen** and **Molly**). Pet forms of Maire include *Maille*, *Mailse*, *Mailti* and the elaboration *Mariona*. *Marie*, pronounced with a long 'a', with the stress on the first syllable rather than in the French way, is also very common in Ireland. *Mari* and *Mairie* are also used. Among the name's Irish holders, one who stands out was Maire Rua Ni Mhathuna (c.1615–86). Rua means 'the red', a reference to her flaming hair. She was the daughter of a chieftain of the O'Mahonys of Co. Clare, had three husbands, and at least nine children. These did not stop her leading an active life, and at one point she was acquitted of the murder of an English settler whose stock she had been raiding.

## Mairead *Mairéad* f.

The Irish form of *Margaret*. Like **Maire** it has been very popular and so has developed many forms, including *Maighread*, *Maighréad*, *Mairéad*, *Maired*, *Mairghréad*, *Maraid*, *Muirád*, *Muirghead*, *Muráid*, and *Muraod*. Peg and Peggy, the English pet forms of Margaret, appear in Irish as *Peig* and *Peigí* with their own pet form *Peigín*, anglicized as *Pegeen*.

## Mairie *see* Maire

## Mairin, Máirín *see* Maureen

## Máirtín *m.*

This is the Irish form of the name *Martin*, originally from a Roman name meaning 'belonging to the god Mars'. Its use spread world-wide in memory of the fourth-century soldier–saint Martin of Tours. *Martán* is an older form of the name.

## Maitiú *m.*

This is the Irish form of *Matthew*, a biblical name meaning 'gift of God'. *Matha* is an older Irish form.

## Majella *f.*

The popularity of St Gerard Majella (1726–55), patron saint of mothers and childbirth, probably influenced the use in Ireland of the name **Gerard**, and parents of girls have adopted his pleasant-sounding surname as an unusual first name.

## Malachy *m.*

Malachy is a name with two sources. One is the name *Maeleachlainn* or *Maoilseachlann* (also *Máelechlainn*, anglicized as *Melaghlin*), meaning 'devotee of St Sechnall or Secundinus' (one of St **Patrick**'s first companions). It was borne by the High King Malachy (949–1022), a husband of **Gormlaith**, who defeated the Vikings at the Battle of Tara in 980 and then re-took Dublin from the Norse invaders. The other source is the reformer St Malachy of Armagh (1094–1148) who helped reorganize the Church in Ireland after the disruptions of the Viking raids. His name was *Maolmaodhog* (earlier Máel Máedóc), meaning 'devotee of Maedoc'. *Máedóc* or *Maodhóg* is a pet form of **Aodh**, and the name of St Maedoc of Ferns (d. 626), who lived in great austerity and is said to have recited 500 psalms a day. Maolmaodhog is also the probable source of the name **Marmaduke**. These names were anglicized as Malachy because of the similarity of sound to Malachi, the biblical prophet whose name means 'my messenger'.

## Malcolm *see* Colm

## Mallaidh *see* Molly

## Malone m.

An Irish surname used as a first name. Its original Irish form, Mael Eoin, means 'servant of (St) John'.

## Mannix *Mainchín* m.

This name is a pet form of the word *manach*, 'monk'. The seventh-century saint known as St *Munchin* the Wise (also found as *Mainchin* and *Manchen*) represents one anglicization of the name, but Mannix is now more common. The use of the English word 'monk' as a first name is to be found in the Irish poet Monk Gibbon.

## Manus *Mánus* m.

Manus has travelled a long way to reach Ireland. It began at the court of Frankish king and emperor Charlemagne (747–814), whose name is a French form of the words 'Charles the Great'. The most famous leader in western Europe, it was thanks to his fame that the simple Frankish name *Charles*, meaning 'man', developed forms in almost every

Western language. Charles the Great translated
into Latin becomes Carolus Magnus, and when
the stories of Charlemagne reached Scandinavia,
the first part of the name became Carl, and the
second was adopted as *Magnus*. This was taken
to Ireland by the Vikings and adopted by the Irish
as Manus. The name's Irish form can also be spelt
*Maghnus*. Of the name's many holders, one of
the most prominent was Manus O'Donnell
(c.1490–1563) chieftain, scholar and poet, who
fought with the Geraldines and O'Neills against
the English, wrote a well-known life of St
*Columba* (see **Colm**) and whose reputation for
wit still lives on in the folklore of Donegal.

## Maodhóg *see* Malachy

## Maoilseachlann *see* Lanty, Malachy

## Maolíosa *m. and f.*

Maolíosa means 'devotee of Jesus' and was well
used from early times. It has been anglicized as
*Maelisa*. It has been a male name for most of its
history, but because it sounds like the girl's name
Melissa (from the Greek for 'bee'), it has also
developed in modern times into a girl's name,
often actually using the form *Melissa*.

**Maolmaodhog** *see* **Malachy**

**Maolmhuire, Maolra, Maolruaní** *see* **Milo**

**Maraid, Margaret** *see* **Mairead**

**Mari, Marie, Mariona** *see* **Maire**

**Marmaduke** *m.*

Marmaduke seems to be an Irish export. While the origin of the name is not entirely certain, the best explanation seems to be that it is a form of the name Mael Maedoc (see **Malachy**). The Vikings and Irish intermarried, and they also exchanged names, the Vikings giving Ireland **Manus** and **Lochlann**, while **Niall** became Njal in Iceland, and the name of the thoroughly Icelandic hero of one of the great Icelandic sagas. It is known from archaeology and dialect and place-name studies that after the Dublin Vikings were expelled from Ireland, they crossed the Irish Sea and settled in certain parts of the north of England, the home-area of Marmaduke being one.

**Martán, Martin** *see* **Máirtín**

**Mary** *see* **Maire**

**Matha** *see* **Maitiú**

## Mathghamhain, Mathúin *see* Mahon

## Matthew *see* Maitiú

## Maura *f.*

Maura is a form of **Maire** which has developed a life of its own. It is being moderately well used in the USA at the moment. Although often spelt *Moira* or *Moyra*, Maura is its usual form in Ireland.

## Maureen *Máirín f.*

This is one of the pet forms of **Maire** which has developed as an independent name. It is also found as *Mairin*, *Maurene* and *Maurine* and in Scotland, *Moirean*. It can be shortened to *Mo*. Technically **Moreen** is a different name, but it is unlikely that many users, at least outside Ireland, distinguish between the two. (See also **Muireann**.)

## Maurice *see* Muiris

## Mave, Meadhbh *see* Maeve

## Meaghan *see* Megan

## Meave, Meaveen *see* Maeve

## Megan *f.*

Megan is a Welsh, not an Irish name, and a pet form of *Margaret*. The only reason for including

this outsider in a book of Irish names is that
many users seem either to think it is Irish or want
it to look like an Irish name. It is very popular in
Canada, Australia and particularly the USA, and
in these countries often appears in imitation-Irish
spellings, such as *Meghan*, *Meaghan* or *Meghann*.

## Meibh, Meidhbhín *see* Maeve

## Melaghlin *see* Malachy

## Melissa *see* Maoilíosa

## Meriel *see* Muirgheal

## Merna *see* Myrna

## Meryl *see* Muirgheal

## Michael *Micheál m.*

Michael is a biblical name meaning 'Who is like
the Lord?' Not widely used until comparatively
modern times, it became so well used that the
Irish short form *Mick* became a slang term for an
Irishman. Its popularity has been enhanced by the
fame of IRA leader Michael Collins (1890–1922),
while the actor Micheál MacLiammóir (1899-1978)
shows the use of the Irish form of the name.

## Milo *m.*

Milo is an Irish development of the name *Miles* or *Myles*. These names were used to translate three native Irish names: *Maeleachlainn* (see **Malachy**); *Maolruaní* (also anglicized as *Mulroney*), 'servant of a champion'; and particularly *Maolra* (earlier *Maolmhuire*), 'devotee of Mary'. Both Myles and Milo are well used in Ireland today, the former well known from Myles na Gopaleen which, along with **Flann** O'Brien, was one of the pen-names of **Brian** O'Nolan (1911–66). The latter name became widely known through the actor Milo O'Shea.

**Mo** *see* **Maureen**

**Moira** *see* **Maura**

**Moirean** *see* **Maureen**

**Móirín** *see* **Moreen**

**Molaise, Molaisse** *see* **Laserian**

## Molly *Mallaidh f.*

This is another pet form of **Maire**. Although by no means restricted to Ireland, it came to be thought of as a typically Irish name, hence its appearance in song and story, such as *Cockles and Mussels* and in Joyce's *Ulysses*. Poll and Polly, developments of Molly, appear in Irish as *Pal*, *Pails* and *Paili*.

## Mona *Muadhnait f.*

In Ireland, Mona is a form of *Muadhnait*, 'noble, good' which has also been anglicized as *Monat*. Elsewhere it can have other sources: either as a pet form of Monica; as an Arab name; or more recently from the old Italian form of Madonna, 'Lady', through a misunderstanding of the title of Leonardo da Vinci's painting *Mona Lisa*.

## Monenna, Moninne *see* Blinne

## Mor *Mór f.*

This name, meaning 'tall, great', was easily the most popular name in late-medieval Ireland. In Scotland, where it was also used, it developed the pet form *Morag*, but its Irish pet form is **Moreen**.

## Morainn, Morann *see* Muireann

## Moreen *Móirín f.*

Moreen is the pet form of **Mor**, 'great, tall', although in practice it is probably freely interchanged with **Maureen**. (See also **Muireann**.)

## Morna *see* Myrna

**Morrin** *see* **Muireann**

**Morris** *see* **Muiris**

**Mortimer** *see* **Murtagh**

**Moyra** *see* **Maura**

**Muadhnait** *see* **Mona**

**Muirád, Muirghead** *see* **Mairead**

**Muircheartach** *see* **Murtagh**

**Muireadhach** *see* **Murry**

## Muireann *Muirinn f.*
This name, which means 'sea-white' or 'sea-fair', is common in myth and legend. Among its holders was the nurse of the hero Cael, who composed a poem for him that won him the bride of his choice; and the wife of **Ossian**. It is also found as *Morrin*, and as *Morann* or *Morainn* in Scotland. Not surprisingly there is a good deal of confusion between this name, and **Maureen** and **Moreen**.

## Muirgheal *f.*
Forms of this name, which means 'sea-bright', occur all the Celtic languages. It is not clear which

one is the original source of *Muriel* and its variants, such as *Meryl* and *Meriel*; probably all played a part. Certainly it has been anglicized as Muriel, and as *Murel* in Ireland. It is also found as *Muiríol*.

## Muirinn *see* Muireann

## Muiríoch *see* Murry

## Muiríol *see* Muirgheal

## Muiris *m.*

This name is the Irish form of *Maurice* or *Morris*. First introduced by the Normans, it is common in Ireland today. It was used in honour of St Maurice and his companions, Christian Roman legionaries who were martyred in about 287 for refusing to sacrifice to the Roman gods. The legionaries had been recruited in Egypt, and Maurice means 'a Moor'. Maurice was also used in Ireland to translate *Muiríos*, an early name meaning 'sea-strength' and **Murrough**, and the popularity of Muiris may be as a re-translation of these uses.

## Muirne *see* Myrna

## Mulroney *see* Milo

**Munchin** *see* **Mannix**

**Mundy** *see* **Redmond**

**Muráid, Muraod** *see* **Mairead**

**Murchadh** *see* **Murrough**

**Murel, Muriel** *see* **Muirgheal**

**Murphy** *m. and f.*
This Irish surname comes from a first name meaning 'hound (i.e. warrior) of the sea'. It has since been readopted as an occasional first name. A rash of female Murphys can be expected after the success of American TV series *Murphy Brown*.

**Murray** *see* **Murry**

**Murrough** *Murchadh m.*
This name, which means 'sea-fighter', was borne by the eldest son of **Brian** Boru, who led his father's troops at the Battle of Clontarf in 1014 where, despite the defeat of the Vikings, they both fell. According to legend, Murrough was able to fight with a sword in each hand. At Clontarf, it is said, he fought so fiercely that his sword became red-hot and its handle melted, making him throw

the sword aside. As a result he was mortally wounded, and died the next sunrise.

## Murry *Muiríoch* m.

Primarily known as a Scottish first name and surname, Murry is also used in Ireland. It means either 'seaman' or 'lord, master'. The name is also found as *Muireadhach* in Irish and as *Murray* in its anglicized form. It was the name of a grandson of **Niall** of the Nine Hostages (Niall Naoi-ghiallach) who was captured as a youth by a Scots king. He escaped, bringing with him a maiden called *Earc*. When a jealous rival killed Muireadhach, Earc revived him by placing in his mouth a herb she had once seen a weasel use to revive her dead mate.

## Murtagh *Muircheartach* m.

This name, meaning 'skilled in seacraft', was very common in early times. In Connacht it becomes **Briartach**, and can also be anglicized as *Murt*, *Murty* or *Murtha*. It was translated *Mortimer*. The semi-mythical Muircheartach Mac Earca was said to be high king of Ireland in the early sixth century. He was the son of Muireadhach and *Earc* (see **Murry**), and the strange tale of his death, torn between the commands of the Church and the allure of a magical lady who persuaded him to abandon his family, is an interesting reflection of the struggle that must have gone on at this time between the forces of paganism and Christianity.

## Myles *see* Milo

## Myrna *Muirne f.*
This was the name of the mother of **Finn** Mac Cool. It also occurs as *Morna* and *Merna*. Myrna gained world-wide fame as the name of the American actress Myrna Loy (1905–93).

# n

**Náble, Náible** *see* **Nápla**

**Naithí** *see* **Dáithi**

**Nano, Nanno** *see* **Nora**

**Naoise** *m.*
Naoise was the man with whom **Deirdre** fell in love, and who was treacherously put to death by Conchobhar Mac Nessa (see **Conor**). The meaning of the name is not known. In the past it was anglicized as *Nyce*, and translated Noah.

**Naomhán** *see* **Nevan**

**Nápla** *f.*
This is an Irish form of *Annabelle*. No one is sure where Annabelle comes from, but one theory is that it is a form of the name Amabel, from the Latin for 'likeable, amiable'. The Normans introduced it

in forms such as Anable or Anaple, which in Irish became *Annábla*. From this, shorter forms such as Nápla, *Náble* or *Náible* became popular.

**Nathí, Nathy** *see* **Dáithí**

**Naugher, Noghor, Nohor** *see* **Conor**

**Neal, Neale** *see* **Niall**

**Néamh** *see* **Niamh**

**Neas** *see* **Eneas**

**Neásan** *see* **Nessan**

**Neassa** *see* **Nessa**

**Neece, Neese, Niece** *see* **Aengus**

**Neil** *see* **Niall**

**Neila, Neilla** *see* **Nelda**

**Neilie, Neilus** *see* **Cornelius**

**Neill, Néill** *see* **Niall**

### Nelda *f.*
This is a modern feminine form of the name **Niall**. *Neila* and *Neilla* have also been used.

### Nelson *see* **Niall**

### Nessa *Neassa f.*
In myth, Nessa was the mother of Conchobhar Mac Nessa (see **Conor**). She was a powerful and ambitious woman who used her attractiveness to promote her son's interests, and thus her own. She was married to **Fachnan**, King of Ulster (though his druid Cathbad was reputed to be Conchobhar's father), and when, after Fachnan's death, his half-brother and heir **Fergus** wanted to marry her, she would only agree to do so if Fergus agreed to let Conchobhar rule for a year. Under Nessa's guidance Conchobhar ruled so well that the people chose him to be their permanent king. Nessa as a first name can also be a pet form of *Agnes* or a short form of **Vanessa**.

### Nessan *Neásan m.*
This name's meaning is unknown, although 'stoat' has been suggested. It was borne by several Irish saints, including St Nessan the Deacon (d. 551), founder of the Mungret monastery near Limerick.

## Nevan *Naomhán* m.

Nevan means 'holy' and was the name of an Irish saint. There is also a surname **Nevin**, formerly Knavin, which has a different source, probably coming from the word for 'bone'. The occasional use of Nevin and Nevan as first names in the USA is more likely to derive from the surname.

## Nia *see* Niamh

## Niall m.

This is the main Irish form of the name more commonly spelt *Neil* or *Neal*. The spelling Neil is also well used in Ireland, and there is an alternative Irish spelling *Néill*; others include *Neale*, *Neill*, *Nial* and *Niel*. In Ireland all forms except Néill are pronounced the same, to sound like 'kneel', but elsewhere Niall is sometimes pronounced to sound like 'Nye-al'. The name's meaning is unclear, but this may be because its form has changed. Its most famous holder was Niall Naoi-ghiallach ('of the Nine Hostages'), and one theory is that his name was originally Nél, meaning 'cloud', but that it was changed to have the same vowel sound as his title, Naoi-ghiallach. Niall was a fifth-century king, but his story has had so many mythical elements added that it is often difficult to separate truth from fiction. The reason he was called 'of the Nine Hostages' was that he was so powerful that many important people gave him hostages for their good behaviour; but the story that he also took hostages from neighbouring countries cannot be true. His raids abroad were probably confined to Britain, and in one of them he may have taken St **Patrick** as a slave. Niall may have been half Romano–British, as his mother was reputedly a British slave called *Cairenn*, which would be the Irish form of the Latin name Carina, or 'beloved'. There is an Irish pet form of Niall, *Niallán*, and the surname-turned-first-name, *Nelson*, was originally 'Neil-son'. Originally used as a first name in honour of the hero of the Battle of Trafalgar (1805), its use has increased lately, particularly among Black Americans, out of respect for South African leader Nelson Mandela. Surprisingly, *Nigel* is also a form of Niall. When medieval scribes, working in Latin, wrote Niall they gave it the form Nigellus, as if it came from the Latin word *niger*, 'black'. When interest was strong in things medieval in the nineteenth century, this form was adopted as Nigel.

## Niamh *f.*

Originally a term for a goddess, this popular name means 'radiance, brightness'. Among those in myth who bore it was Niamh of the Golden Hair, daughter of Manannán, the sea god. She fell in love with **Finn**'s son **Ossian** and they went to the Land of Promise. Enchanted, he thought he had stayed three weeks, but later found it had been three hundred years. The actress Niamh Cusack has brought it to a wider audience. *Nia*, the Welsh form, can be found in the USA (although there it is also used as a name from Swahili) and the old Irish name *Néamh* is probably another form. Niamh is currently very popular in Ireland.

## Niel, Nigel *see* Niall

## Noel *Nollaig* m., Noelle *Nollaig* f.

This name's Irish form is the word 'Christmas'. For no known reason it was a hugely popular name in Ireland in the earlier twentieth century, and used far more often than there were Christmas babies born. It is fairly unusual for an Irish word in having the same form in the masculine and feminine.

## Nóinín, Nóirín *see* Nora

## Nola *see* Nuala

## Nolan *m.*

This Irish surname is surprisingly well used as a first name in the USA, as in the baseball player

Nolan Ryan. It comes from *nuall,* meaning 'shout'.
It is also found as *Noland* and *Nolen*.

## Noleen *see* Nuala

## Nolen *see* Nolan

## Nollaig *see* Noel

## Nora *Nóra*, Noreen *Nóirín f.*

These are the two most common of the names
that were originally pet forms of *Onóra* (see
**Honor**), although few users would still connect
these names. Other pet forms of Onóra include
*Nonie* (also used for **Siobhan**), *Nano*, *Nanno*,
*Norlene* and *Nóinín*, the Irish for 'daisy'. Noreen is
also spelt *Norene* or *Norine*, and Nora can appear
as *Norah* or its American elaboration, *Norita*.

## Nuala *f.*

Nuala is a short form of *Fionnuala* (see **Finola**),
'fair or white shoulder'. Recently a popular name,
it is probably used more widely than the full form.
*Nola* is an alternative, and there is a pet form,
*Noleen*.

## Nyce *see* Naoise

# O

**Odanodan** *see* **Adamnan**

**Odharnait** *see* **Orna**

**Odhrán, Odrán** *see* **Oran**

**Óengus** *see* **Aengus**

**Oghe, Oghie, Oho** *see* **Eochaidh**

**Oilbhe** *see* **Alby**

**Oilibhéar** *m.*
This is the Irish form of *Oliver*, a form of the
Scandinavian Olaf, 'heir to his ancestors'. It was
taken into the body of Irish names directly from
the Vikings as *Amhlaoibh* (see **Auliffe**). The form
Oilibhéar came into use via the Normans, who
would have brought with them the name's French
form, Olivier. After Oliver Cromwell's Irish

atrocities use of the name stopped, but it recovered with the beatification of Oliver Plunket (1625–81), the bishop of Armagh martyred after Titus Oates' infamous Popish Plot. He was canonized in 1976.

**Oisín** *see* **Ossian**

**Oistín** *see* **Augusteen**

**Olaf, Olave** *see* **Auliffe**

**Oliver** *see* **Oilibhéar**

**Onan** *see* **Adamnan**

**Onóra** *see* **Honor, Nora**

**Oona, Oonagh** *see* **Una**

### Oran *Odhrán* m.

Oran comes from a word meaning 'grey-brown, dark', and is the masculine equivalent of **Orna**. It is also found as *Órán* and *Odrán*. There were seventeen saints Oran, but little of certainty is known of them and their stories tend to get confused. One who stands out is St Oran of Iona, who may have built the first church on the island, even before the arrival of *Columba* (see **Colm**).

His chapel there is still venerated. In the USA
*Orin* or *Orrin* (also spelt *Or(r)en* or *Orran*) is
quite a common name, and is most probably a
development of Oran. It has also been quite well
used in literature, featuring in Raymond Chandler's
*The Little Sister* (1949) and Eugene O'Neill's
*Mourning Becomes Electra* (1931). Oran is
increasingly popular in Ireland.

### Órfhlaith *see* Orla

### Orin *see* Oran

### Orinthia *f.*

This unusual and rather pretty name qualifies as
Irish only in that it was invented by an Irishman,
George Bernard Shaw, for his play *The Apple Cart*
(1929). Attempts have been made to link it with
**Oran**, but it is more likely to be pure invention.
Shaw had a liking for new or unusual names for
his heroines – Jennifer and Candida, for instance,
were very rare until he gave them publicity.

### Orla *Órla f.*

This name means 'golden lady'. Although popular
in the Middle Ages, it does not, surprisingly, seem
to have belonged to a saint or to a notable person
in myth. It has been well used in the last twenty-

five years and has spread to the USA. It is occasionally found in the earlier forms *Órfhlaith* and *Orlaith*; *Orlagh* is a common variant, and it can also be found as *Aurnia* and even *Orley*.

### Orna *Odharnait f.*

This is the feminine version of **Oran**, meaning 'grey-brown, dark'. In the anglicized form the final 't' is missing, probably to match the model of **Orla**.

## Orran, Orrin, Or(r)en *see* Oran

## Oscar *Osgar m.*

This is probably the most recent of many names exchanged between Ireland and Scandinavia (e.g. see **Marmaduke**). So popular has it been in Scandinavia, particularly Sweden, that some books on first names even give it a meaning derived from Germanic roots, but the name is indubitably Irish, meaning 'deer lover'. In legend Oscar was the son of **Ossian** and the grandson of **Finn**, and his personality reflected his ancestry. He was the mightiest warrior in his generation of the Fianna, the traditional royal bodyguard. With his grandfather apparently dead, and his father with **Niamh** in the Land of Promise, Oscar was leader of the Fianna; but the new king, **Cairbre**, wanted to get rid of them. In a great battle at Gabhra

(traditionally Garristown, Co. Dublin), Oscar
killed Cairbre, but was himself mortally wounded.
His death ended the stories of the Fenian Cycle.
The Scottish poet James Macpherson made Oscar
the hero of some of his *Ossian* poems. They had
enormous success across Europe, where use of
the name spread. One admirer of the poems was
Napoleon Bonaparte, who carried a copy on
campaign with him. When his Marshal Jean-
Baptiste Bernadotte had his first son, Napoleon
was godfather and gave the boy the name Oscar.
Bernadotte later received greater promotion, for
Napoleon made him king of Sweden, and the boy
succeeded his father to become Oscar I of Sweden.
It became a traditional name in the royal house
and soon spread throughout Scandinavia. In turn,
Oscar I's court physician was the world-renowned
Irish ophthalmologist, Sir William Wilde. His wife,
Lady Jane Wilde, was a nationalist and poet. With
such a background, it was not surprising that their
son was christened Oscar Fingal O'Flahertie
Wills Wilde. Oscar Wilde's notorious trials for
homosexuality in 1895 made the name unusable
for several generations, and it is only now coming
back into use. However, in the USA, with a large
number of immigrants from both Ireland and
Sweden, it never lost favour, and it is moderately

popular there at the moment both as Oscar and in the Scandinavian spelling *Oskar*.

## Osheen *see* Ossian

## Oskar *see* Oscar

## Ossian *Oisín* m.

*Osheen* or *Ossin* are probably better anglicizations of Oisín, but thanks to the poems of James Macpherson Ossian is the best-known form of the name. There are many, often conflicting, stories told of Ossian, but all agree that he was the son of **Finn** Mac Cool. One version of Ossian's birth says that **Sive**, his beautiful mother, was turned into a deer by the Dark Druid. She fled into the forest where she gave birth to her son. Several years later Finn was out hunting in the forest and found a handsome little boy who told him he had been raised by a deer. Finn realized this must be his son, and called him Oisín, 'little deer'. Ossian had a great reputation as a poet and for his wisdom, but this did not prevent his going to the Land of Promise with **Niamh**. When he returned three hundred years had passed and as soon as Ossian's foot touched Irish soil he became an old, old man. It was in this form that he met St **Patrick** and was, we are told, converted by him. The debate between Ossian and Patrick which led to his conversion became a popular literary form, new versions being written until at least the eighteenth century. The sculptor Oisin Kelly (1915–81), whose work can be seen in many Irish churches, was one modern holder of the name. Oisin is a popular choice in Ireland at the moment.

### Ounan *see* Adamnan

### Owen *see* Eoghan, Eoin

### Owny *Uaithne* m. and f.

This name means 'greenish', and can be used for both sexes, although it is more often masculine, with *Uaine* being used for the feminine. It was the name of Owny MacRory O'More, son of the great **Rory** Oge O'More. Like his father he was an incessant fighter against the English, and was eventually killed in a skirmish at Timahoe in 1600, but only after he had recovered most of Leix. The name is also spelt *Uaitne* and anglicized as *Owney*, *Oynie* and *Hewney*, and in the past could even be translated literally into English as Green.

### Oyne, Oynie *see* Eoghan, Owny

# p

**pa, paddy, padhra, pádhraic, pádhraig, pádraic** *see* **patrick**

**pádraigín** *see* **patricia**

**páid, paidí, páidi, páidín** *see* **patrick**

**paili, pails** *see* **molly**

**paití** *see* **patricia, patrick**

**pal** *see* **molly**

**páraic, parra** *see* **patrick**

**parthalan** *parthalán* m.
This is an Irish form of the biblical *Bartholomew*, which was given to a mythical early settler of Ireland. St *Jerome* wrongly interpreted Bartholomew to mean 'son of him who stays the water', which

must have led to the name's association with
Noah, for Parthalan is described as the leader of
the first people to occupy Ireland after Noah's
flood. This is an old tradition, recorded as early as
the ninth century. But Parthalan's settlement was
eventually struck by a plague, and all or all but
one of the settlers died. The name is still used
today and occurs in a wide range of spellings,
including *Parthalón*, *Pártlán*, *Párthlán*, *Partnán*,
*Partlón* and *Beartlaidh*. Its anglicizations include
**Barclay** and its variants, *Parlan* and, perhaps most
frequently at the moment, *Bartley* and *Batt*.

## Pat *see* Patricia, Patrick

## Patricia *f.*
Although a feminine form of **Patrick** and current
in Ireland, Patricia is an international name rather
than an Irish one. It is said, on no very strong
evidence, to have appeared first in Scotland in the
eighteenth century (although as a Roman name
it existed earlier, there being a seventh-century
St Patricia of Naples), and did not become common
in Ireland until the twentieth century. The form
Patricia is used in English, French, Spanish and
Portuguese, and appears as Patrizia in Italy. *Pat* and
*Patty* are short forms, but in Ireland *Patsy* is still
used as a masculine form, although it is feminine

elsewhere. The Irish feminine form of Patrick, *Pádraigín*, is also modern, only becoming well-used in the twentieth century. Its pet form is *Paití*.

## Patrick *Pádraig* m.

It need hardly be said that St Patrick is the patron saint of Ireland. Despite the existence of his autobiography, it is still difficult to sift out hard fact from the vast amount of myth that surrounds him. He is thought to have lived from about 373 to 463, but even that is much disputed. His name, Roman in origin, means 'noble', and it is known from his own writings that he was British, the son of a town councillor and deacon, and the grandson of a priest. He was captured as a youth by Irish raiders – perhaps those of **Niall** of the Nine Hostages – and spent six years as a slave in Ireland, during which time he had a vision urging him to convert his captors. After escaping from slavery he eventually made his way to the Continent where he trained as a priest. His life and myth become hopelessly mixed after his return to Ireland, but there is no doubt that by the time he died a considerable part of the country was converted (not all, of course, directly by Patrick). Because of the awe in which the saint was held, his name was very little used in Ireland before the seventeenth century, but since at least the nineteenth it has been one of the country's most popular names. Because of this it appears in a bewildering variety of forms, including *Pádraic*, *Pádhraig*, *Pádhraic*, *Phadrig*, *Phaedrig* and *Páraic*, with pet forms *Padhra*, *Páid*, *Páidi*, *Paidí*, *Paití*, *Páidín*, *Parra* and *Paudeen*. Anglicized pet forms include *Pa*, *Pat* and *Patsy*. The most popular pet form in Ireland is *Paddy*, but it needs to be used with care, as its use outside Ireland as a general term for an Irishman is often felt by the Irish to be racist and offensive. Patrick has also been very popular in France, where it has almost replaced Patrice, the name's French form.

### Patsy *see* Patricia, Patrick

### Patty *see* Patricia

### Paudeen *see* Patrick

### Paul *see* Pól

### Peadar *m.*
The modern Irish form of *Peter*, 'the rock'. It is also found as *Peadair*. Older forms are listed at **Pierce**.

### Pearce *see* Pierce

**Degeen, Deig, Deigí(n)** *see* **Mairead**

**Derce, Derse** *see* **Dierce**

**Deter** *see* **Feoras, Deadar, Dierce**

**Dhadrig, Dhaedrig** *see* **Datrick**

**Dhelan** *see* **Felan**

**Dhelim** *Feidhlim* m.
Phelim or *Felim* is an ancient name of obscure
meaning. It can also appear as *Feidhlimidh*,
and among the historical holders of the name
was Feidhlimidh Mac Criomhthainn (770–847),
King of Munster. He was also a lay member of a
community of monks called the Companions of
God and is said to have been bishop of Cashel.
However, he also seems to have been a highly
successful warrior, and a strange mixture of the
religious and the secular. This mix is illustrated in
the story that when he lost a battle to a rival king
he fled the field, leaving his crosier behind.
Another holder of the name was Phelim MacFiach
O'Byrne (see **Fiach** for his father), who defeated
the English at Glenmalure, Co. Wicklow, in 1599.
The name is also anglicized as *Phelimy*, *Felimy*
and *Felimid*.

## Philip *see* Pilib

## Philomena *f.*

In 1802 a tomb bearing an inscription interpreted as meaning 'Peace be with you, Philomena' was found in the catacombs of Rome. The tomb held the bones of a girl of about fifteen years, and a phial of blood. Within a few years St Philomena's cult sprang up, miracles were reported at her tomb and the pope officially recognized the cult in 1835. But scholars cast doubt on her existence, and the cult was suppressed in 1960. However, she still has her defenders. And the inscription? Philomena means 'beloved', and the Latin is now interpreted simply as 'Rest in peace, Beloved'. It was a popular name in Ireland in the first half of the twentieth century, but use fell away after her cult's suppression. The name is also spelt *Phylomena*, and the occurrence in Ireland of the rare name *Philomela*, the woman who in Greek myth was turned into a nightingale, may be due to the similarity in sound.

## Pierce *Piaras m.*

Pierce is another Irish form of the name *Peter*. While **Peadar** is a modern form taken directly from Peter, the Irish had much earlier adopted the

French form Piers, brought over by the Normans.
This became both **Feoras** and *Piaras* in Irish, and
is also found in the forms *Pearce*, *Perce* and *Perse*.
The actor Pierce Brosnan is a well-known bearer.

## Pilib *m.*

This is the Irish form of the name *Philip*, 'lover of
horses', which has been used since Norman times.

## Pól *m.*

Pól is the Irish form of the name *Paul*, which
comes from the Latin word for 'small'. It has only
been popular in Ireland in modern times.

## Proinsias *m.*, Proinséas *f.*

These are the Irish forms of *Francis* and *Frances*.
These names come from St Francis of Assisi, who
was christened Giovanni, but got his more familiar
name as a nickname meaning 'little Frenchman'
from his love of fashionable French things in
his youth. There is a pet form of Proinsias,
*Preanndaigh*, sometimes translated *Frank*, and
*Proinseasa* (Francesca) can be translated Frankie.
Both the masculine and feminine forms of the
name can also be spelt *Proinnsias*.

# q

**Quentin** *see* **Quintin**

**Queran** *see* **Kieran**

**Quinlan** *Caoinleán* m.
Caoinleán means 'of beautiful shape', and is the
source of the surnames *Quilan* and *Quinlevan*,
both of which have been used as first names.

**Quinn** m.
This Irish surname is used as a boy's first name,
particularly in the USA. As a surname it can have
two sources, either the name **Conn**, probably
meaning 'sense, intelligence', or *Coinneach*,
'pleasant person' (see under **Canice**). Quinn can
also be a short form of **Quintin**, or of Quincy,
which comes from a Norman place-name.

# Quintin *m.*

This is really an English name, taken from various place-names meaning 'queen's town'; but in Ireland it has been used to anglicize *Cúmháí* (earlier *Cú Mhaighe*). This name means 'hound of the plain', the term 'hound' in Irish often implying 'warrior'. Cúmhaí was also anglicized as *Quinton*, *Quentin* and *Cooey*. Quinton is currently rather popular in the USA where, as well as Quintin and Quentin, it is also found as *Quinnton*, *Quintan*, *Quinten* and *Quintyn*.

# R

### Raghnailt *f.*

This feminine form of **Randal** is one of the girl's names borrowed by the Irish from the Vikings. Far fewer of these seem to have survived than of the masculine borrowings. It is also found in Scots Gaelic as *Raghnaid*, and it is possible that this is the source of the name *Rhona* (but see **Ronan**). In Latin documents Raghnailt becomes *Regina*, and this was sometimes used to translate the name.

### Raghnall *see* Randal

### Raidhrí *see* Rory

### Ranait *see* Ronit

### Randal *Raghnall m.*

Another Irish borrowing from the Vikings, this is the masculine form of **Raghnailt**. In modern

Scandinavian languages the name is Ragnvald, and is made up of elements meaning 'advice, decision' and 'ruler'. In English the name is Ronald. There is a modern Irish form **Raonull** and it can also be anglicized as **Ranald** or **Rannal**. **Rynal** is probably another anglicization. Randal is also used for **Rannulbh**, in modern English Randolph, or 'shield-wolf'. Randal MacDonnel, Earl of Antrim (d. 1636), occupied an uneasy position between the Irish and English. He was the son of **Sorley** Boy MacDonnell, so was of mixed Irish and Scottish descent. He had joined the Irish rebellion of 1600, but on becoming head of his house submitted to England, and was rewarded by being made first Earl of Antrim. His co-operation with the English did not make him popular, and a few years later he survived an attempt to remove him as head of his house.

## Raymond *see* Redmond

## Reagan *m.*
This surname, usually **Regan** in Ireland, is occasionally found as a first name. It comes either from *rí*, 'king', or from *ríodhgach*, 'impulsive, furious'.

## Réamann, Reamon *see* Redmond

## Rearden *see* Riordan

## Redmond *Réamann* m.

Redmond is the Irish form of the Germanic name that occurs in modern English as **Raymond**. There is debate as to whether it comes from the old English form of the name or from the Norman, but they were very similar, and both came from two elements meaning 'advice or counsel' and 'protection'. It is also found as **Reamon**, and **Mundy** is said to be a short form. The name is quite widely used and is traditional in the O'Hanlon family. One Redmond O'Hanlon (Réamonn Ó hAnluain, d. 1681) was a notorious highwayman and charismatic outlaw in Ulster and north Leinster for seven years, leading a band of about fifty followers who made most of their money by raising a 'black rent' (extortion) from English planters and other wealthy people. Less than a century after his death there was already enough lore attached to his name for a thrilling popular book to be written of his life. Redmond O'Hanlon has a modern namesake who is a well-known travel writer.

## Regan *see* Reagan

## Regina *see* Raghnailt, Ríona

**Reidhrí** *see* **Rory**

**Reilly** *see* **Riley**

**Renagh** *see* **Ríona**

**Renny** *see* **Ronit**

**Rhona** *see* **Raghnailt, Ronan**

**Ríain, Rian** *see* **Ryan**

**Ribeard, Ribeart, Ribirt** *see* **Roibéard**

**Richael** *f.*
This pretty and unusual Irish name is said to have been the name of a virgin saint whose feast day is 19 May. It can be anglicized as *Richella*.

**Richard** *see* **Ristéard**

**Riley** *m. and f.*
This form of the Irish surname is enjoying some popularity in the USA, more often as a boy's name, but also as a girl's. The surname in Ireland is more usually *Reilly*, which is also used in the USA, along with *Rylee* and *Ryley*. The name's Irish form is Ó Raghallaigh, from Raghallach, an old Irish name of unknown meaning, although 'valiant' has been suggested.

## Riobart, Riobárt *see* Roibéard

## Riocard *see* Ristéard

### Ríona *f.*

Ríona is a form of the name *Ríonach* (earlier *Ríoghnach*) which means 'queenly'. Not surprisingly, it has been translated *Regina*, which has more or less the same meaning. *Renagh* is probably another form, and the name can also be used as a short form of **Catriona**.

### Riordan *m.*

The name Ríoghbhardáin, meaning 'royal poet', developed into *Ríordáin* which was anglicized as Riordan or *Rearden*. The post of king's poet was an ancient and important one, training for which took may years. It involved learning not only to recite all the traditional stories from heart and composing in the complicated metres of the time, but also a knowledge of legal judgements and local lore and law. In the nineteenth century, when the Irish language was being eroded by concerted English efforts to suppress it, poets helped to keep it going. Despite its meaning, exclusive use of the name for one profession ceased relatively early, and there was a Munster king of the name who died in 1058.

### Ristéard *m.*

This is one of the Irish forms of the name *Richard*, 'strong ruler'. The original English form of the name was Ricard, with a hard 'c', the softer 'ch' form, Richard, being French. Both forms came into Ireland where they became the Irish forms Ristéard, from Richard, and *Riocard*, from Ricard. In the Waterford area Ristéard has become *Risderd*.

### Robert, Robin *see* Roibeard

### Rodan *see* Rowan

### Roden *m.*

This Irish surname from the word *rod*, meaning 'strong', is occasionally used as a first name, especially in the USA. Roden Noel, poet and literary critic, is a holder of the name.

### Roderick *see* Rory

### Rodhlann *m.*

This is the Irish form of the name *Roland*. Roland, coming from elements meaning 'fame' and 'land', was one of the great heroes of early French epics, and the Norman charge at the Battle of Hastings in 1066 was led, according to tradition, by a minstrel singing the *Song of Roland*. When the

Normans in turn invaded Ireland they would have
brought with them both the name of this Roland,
and that of his faithful companion Oliver (see
**Oilibhéar**). There is a pet form, *Rodhlaidhe*.

## Roibeard *m.*

Roibeard is the Irish form of **Robert**, a Germanic
name composed of elements meaning 'fame' and
'bright' (which also implies the sense 'fame'). It
was introduced by the Normans and developed a
number of spellings, including *Roibeárd*, *Ribeard*,
*Ribeart*, *Ribirt*, *Riobárt* and *Riobart*. The pet form
**Robin** has *Roibín* or *Roibean* as its Irish equivalent.

## Roisín *Róisín f.*

The Irish name Róisín is a pet form of **Rós**, in
English, **Rose**. Language experts, who seem to
have no romance in their souls, claim that this
does not derive from the flower name, but is
from a Germanic element *hros*, meaning 'horse'.
However, generations have thought the name
Rose derived from the flower, so in practice that
is what it means. Róisín is usually anglicized as
Roisin or **Rosheen** nowadays, but in the past it
was **Rosaleen**, as in the case of the song *Róisín
Dhu*, which is usually translated 'Dark Rosaleen'.
Róisín Dhu is a poetic symbol of Ireland, and in
the song she is told not to be downhearted, for

her friends are returning from abroad to come to her aid. Because of this, Rosaleen was a popular name in Ireland, either in its original form, or in variants such as *Rosalie* or *Rosaline*. Other more elaborate forms of Rose, such as *Rosanna* (and its variants *Roseanna*, *Rosannah*, *Roseannah*) and *Rosina* are also well used in Ireland, but Roisin or Rosheen remain the most popular forms.

## Roland *see* Rodhlann

## Ronan *Rónán m.*

Ronan is a early name meaning 'little seal' and was borne by up to twelve saints in Ireland and Scotland. However, it tends to be confused with **Rowan** in early records, and it is not always easy to sort out which is which. St Ronan Finn (d. 664) cursed his tormentor, Mad Sweeny (Suibhne Gealt; see also **Sivney**), driving him to madness. A fifth-century St Ronan was said to have been consecrated bishop by St **Patrick**. He worked as a missionary in Brittany and Cornwall, and is buried at Locronan. Another was a seventh-century Scottish hermit who was supposed to have been 'tormented by the evil tongues of the women' of Eoroby on the island of Lewis, and was taken by a whale to the island of North Rona, where he built the chapel whose ruins can still be seen. There is a feminine form of the name, *Rónnad* or *Rónait* (*Ronat*). As St Ronan of North Rona is said by some to have given his name to the island, *Rona* or *Rhona* can also be used as a feminine form of the name. The origin of Rhona is debated. Some would trace it to the island, while others think it is a form of **Raghnailt**.

### Ronit Rathnait f.

Ronit is from the word *rath*, meaning 'prosperity, grace'. It was the name of the patron saint of Kilraghts, Co. Antrim. It can be spelt *Ranait* in Irish and has also been anglicized as *Renny*.

### Rónnad *see* Ronan

### Rory Ruairí m.

Rory comes from the Irish meaning 'red king', but in the past has become confused with the Norse name which gives us *Roderick*, from elements meaning 'fame' and 'ruler', and some older books give this as the name's source. Ruairí is also spelt *Ruaidhrí*, and there are regional variations spelt *Raidhrí* and *Reidhrí*. The name belonged to two outstanding members of the O'More family, Rory O'More (d. c.1555) and his more famous son, Rory Oge O'More of Leix. Rory Oge ('the younger') devoted his life to fighting the English, and scored many runaway successes, but he was finally killed in 1578 and his head displayed at Dublin Castle as a warning to others.

## Rosa *see* Ross

## Rosaleen, Rosalie, Rosaline, Rosanna, Rosannah, Roseanna, Roseannah, Rosheen, Rosina *see* Roisin

## Ross *m.*

Ross is from the word for 'headland'. Although it is thought of nowadays as a mainly Scottish name, it has a long history of use in Ireland. In myth, for example, Ross the Red is supposed to have been the founder of the Red Branch, the warriors who guarded Ulster and had **Cúchulainn** as their greatest champion. In real life an archbishop of Armagh called Ross MacMahon was a leading opponent of Oliver Cromwell. The form of the name *Rosa* probably looks too much like a girl's name to be used today.

## Rowan *Ruan m.* and *f.*

This name comes from *rúad*, 'red', and means 'red-haired man'. It can still be found in Irish in its older spelling of **Ruadhán**. St *Ruadhan* (d. c.548;

also found under the name of *Ruadan* and *Rodan*), founder of the monastery at Lorrha in Co. Tipperary was, according to tradition, a great miracle-worker who saved many lives, but who cursed the royal court at **Tara**, as a result of which Tara was left ruined and deserted. It is doubtful if Rowan as a girl's name is often the same as the boy's. Instead, it is usually thought of as using the alternative name of the beautiful tree, the red-berried mountain ash. It is also used for girls in a form that has the stress on the second syllable rather than the first, as if an elaboration of the name Ann; indeed, it is occasionally found spelt *Rowann* or *Rowanne*. For parents who prefer a genuinely Irish feminine form of Rowan, the name *Rúanhnait* was said to have been borne by the sister of St Rowan.

### Ruaidhrí, Ruairí *see* Rory

### Ruan, Rúanhnait *see* Rowan

### Ryan *Ríain* m.

The meaning of this name is doubtful. It most probably comes from the word *rí*, for 'king', and the most attractive explanation is that it means 'little king'. The name became internationally famous through the success of the actor Ryan

O'Neal in the film *Love Story* in 1970. It is normally used in its basic spelling, but can also be found as *Rian*, *Ryen* and *Ryon*.

**Rylee, Ryley** *see* **Riley**

**Rynal** *see* **Randal**

**Ryon** *see* **Ryan**

# S

**Sabena, Sabia, Sabina, Sabine, Sadhbh, Saidhbhín** *see* **Sive**

**Samhairle** *see* **Sorley**

### Saoirse *f.*
A modern girl's name based on the word for 'freedom', which could be translated Liberty. It is increasingly popular in Ireland.

### Saraid *f.*
Saraid means 'excellent, best'. It was the name of a daughter of **Conn** Céad Cathach ('of the Hundred Battles'), so if his name means 'sense, intelligence', then hers would be a suitable name for his child. Saraid, through marriage, was said to be the ancestress of both the people of Muskerry and of the kings of Scots. Given the similarity of sound, it is not surprising that Saraid was one of the names

translated Sarah. The word *sár*, 'best, noble', occurs in other little-used early-Irish names, such as the girl's name *Sárnait* and its masculine form, *Sárán*.

## Séafraid *m.*

This is an Irish form of *Geoffrey*, and its meaning has been much discussed. There is agreement that the name's second half comes from a Germanic element meaning 'peace' but the source of the first half is obscure. Geoffrey was a popular name with the Normans, who would have taken it to Ireland. It developed a number of forms in two distinct groups, the first under **Seathrún**, while variants of the Séafraid group include *Séafra*, *Siofraidh* and *Séafraidh*. The name was anglicized as *Sheary*.

## Seaghán *see* Sean

## Seamus *Séamas m.*

Seamus or *Shamus* (a particularly American form) is a form of *James*. St James the Great, apostle and martyr, was believed to be buried in Spain at Santiago de Compostela. Particularly from the twelfth to fifteenth centuries, pilgrims flocked from all over Europe to visit his tomb. As a result, there is hardly a European language that does not have a form of his name prominent in its list of national first names. Not surprisingly, there are a number of different spellings, including **Seumas**, **Seumus** and frequently **Séamus**. It is spelt Seumas in Scotland and anglicized as **Hamish**. In Ireland it is also anglicized as **Shemus** and can be shortened to **Shay**. The Irish equivalents of Jimmy are **Séimí**, **Siomaidh** or **Síomaigh**, and **Simidh**, and there are other pet forms, **Séamuisín** and **Siomataigh**. Of the name's many current famous bearers, one of the most respected is Ireland's 1995 Nobel Prize-winning poet, Seamus Heaney.

## Sean **Seán** m.

The Norman invaders brought with them the name Jean, the French form of **John**, and it was this that developed into Sean. John itself is biblical, from the Hebrew name meaning 'the Lord is gracious'. Sean has also been spelt Seón and **Seaghán** and there is a pet form, **Seantaigh**. It is by no means the only form of John in Irish: see also **Eoin**, **Seón**, **Shane** and **Shawn**. Sean has had many famous bearers including, from twentieth-century Irish literature, the playwright Sean O'Casey (1880–1964) and the writer Sean O'Faolain (1900–91). The American actress Sean Young may start a trend for the name's use for girls, just as the variant Shawn is now used in America for both sexes.

### Seanach, Seanán, Seanchán *see* Senan

### Seantaigh *see* Sean

### Séarlait *f.*

This is a relatively recent Irish form of the name *Charlotte*, itself originally a French feminine form of *Charles*. Charlotte was very popular in England in the eighteenth and nineteenth centuries, and the name probably reached Ireland from there.

### Séarlas *m.*

Séarlas, also found in the form *Séarlus*, is an Irish form of *Charles*, itself a Germanic name meaning 'man'. Although it was hardly used in Ireland before the reign of Charles I, it was already an international royal name thanks to the fame of Charlemagne or Charles the Great, Emperor of the Franks, whose name is also the source of **Manus**.

### Seathrún *m.*

This, like **Séafraid** (where the name is discussed more fully) and **Siothrún**, is an Irish form of *Geoffrey*. It is also spelt *Séathrún* and *Searthún*, *Séartha* or *Séarthra*, and can be anglicized as *Sheron*. One of its most famous bearers was Seathrún Céitinn (1580–1644), a priest and scholar who wrote *Foras Feasa ar Eéirinn*, a highly influential four-volume history of Ireland.

## Séimí *see* **Seamus**

## Selia *see* **Sheila**

## Senan *Seanán m.*

This is a name that comes from *sean*, meaning 'old, wise', and ultimately connected with the Latin word which gives the word 'senator'. It would have started life as a nickname, used as a term of respect. St Senan (d. c.544) was a famed founder of monasteries, most notably that on Scattery Island, near Kilrush, Co. Clare, whose ruins can still be seen. Legend states that before he could found it he first had to banish a great monster, combat the local king's claim to the island and defeat the attempts of the king's wizard to expel him. The Irish form of Senan is also spelt *Sionán*, and it has been anglicized as *Sinan*, *Synan*, and *Sinon*. There are two other Irish masculine names from the same root, *Seanach* and *Seanchán*, but these do not seem to be in general use.

## Seoirse *m.*

This is the Irish form of *George*, a name from the Greek meaning 'farmer'. Because of this St George was the patron saint of farmers as well as of soldiers. *Seorsa* is a pet form. The use of the term 'St George's Channel' for the Irish Sea derives from a legend stating that St George, England's patron saint, arrived in that country by sea from the west. Although there are allusions to St George in some early Irish lists of saints, the name was not much used until the Hanoverian period, when four successive Georges held the British throne.

## Seón *m.*

A later form of the name **Sean**, this is, therefore, yet another Irish form of the name *John*.

## Seorsa *see* Seoirse

## Seosaimhín *f.*

This is the Irish form of *Josephine*, a feminine form of *Joseph*. The name is apparently French in origin and certainly became known through the French Empress Josephine, Napoleon's first wife. The Irish is a direct adaptation of the name's English form. Josephine was also used to translate **Siobhan**.

## Seosamh *m.*

This is the Irish version of *Joseph*, a name from the Hebrew meaning 'God shall add (another son)'. Although borne by a great biblical patriarch, in Ireland it is most likely to be used in honour of the husband of the Virgin Mary. It also appears in the forms **Seosap** and **Seosaph**. An earlier form of the name, **Iósep** or **Ióseph**, is equally well used.

## Seumas, Seumus *see* Seamus

## Shaela *see* Shayla

## Shahla *see* Sheila

## Shaila *see* Shayla

## Shain *see* Shane

## Shala *see* Shayla

## Shamus *see* Seamus

## Shana *see* Shanna

## Shane *m.*

This is a northern form of the name **Sean**, an Irish form of *John*. In Ireland its outstanding holder was Shane 'the Proud' O'Neill. He was the son of **Conn** O'Neill, who gave up the chiefly title 'The O'Neill' in return for that of Earl of Tyrone; but Shane rejected all things English. He controlled a vast power base in Ulster from 1558 to 1567. Outside Ireland the name has been spread by a very different route, winning fame from *Shane*, the 1953 classic western film based on the novel by

Jack Schaefer. This, no doubt, is the main source of the name's popularity in the USA, where it is also found in the forms *Shain* and *Shayne*.

## Shanna *f.*

A modern American name which could have various sources, this is most likely a short version of the name **Shannon**, influenced, perhaps, by other Irish names beginning with the sound 'Sha-'. An alternative view is that it is a version of the Irish surname Shannagh, which comes from a first name related to **Senan**. The name has indeed been recorded as *Shannagh*, but this could simply be a spelling device used to make the name look more Irish. It is also found as *Shannah* and *Shana*.

## Shannon *f. and m.*

The name of Ireland's longest river, Shannon has been popular as a first name in the USA for over twenty years but until recently was little used in Ireland itself. Coming from the same root as **Senan**, it means 'the old one'. The river-name was recorded as early as the second century by the Egyptian geographer Ptolemy. Evidence exists across the Celtic world for the recognition of a divine spirit in springs, rivers and lakes, so it seems likely that Shannon is a survival of the name of a pagan god. Well used for girls, it is also

found as a boy's name. In the USA the masculine
form has developed the variants *Shannen* and
*Shanon*, while feminine forms include these and
*Channon*, *Shannyn* or *Shanyn*.

## Shaughan, Shaun, Shauna, Shaunna, Shaunee, Shauni *see* Shawn

### Shavon *f.*

Shavon is the most popular American spelling of
the Irish name **Siobhan**; others include *Shavawn*,
*Shavonn*, *Shavonne*, *Shevon*, *Shivon*, *Shivonne*,
and *Shovon*. As the name's pronunciation is far
from what might be expected by those unfamiliar
with Gaelic, it is not surprising that such phonetic
spellings develop when a name becomes popular.

### Shawn *m. and f.*

Shawn and *Shaun* are phonetic spellings of **Sean**,
one of the Irish forms of *John*. These two forms
have been particularly popular in Britain, while in
the USA there has developed a specifically Black
American form, *DeShawn*. Very occasionally the
name is found as *Shaughan*. Until recently Shawn
and Shaun have been exclusively masculine, but
they are now increasingly used for girls, as with
the Country singer Shawn Colvin. However, more
obviously feminine forms are commoner still,

such as *Shawna* or *Shauna* (also *Shaunna* or
*Shawnna*), and *Shawndelle*, a form which seems
to have developed in Canada. In the USA there is
another group of girl's names where the two
radically different names Shawn and Shawnee,
the latter the name of the Native American nation,
seem to have fallen together to make the new
names *Shaunee*, *Shauni* and *Shawnie*.

### Shay *see* Seamus

### Shay, Shaye *see* Shea

### Shayla *f.*
This is a variant form of the name **Sheila** used in
the USA. Other similar forms found there are
*Shaela*, *Shaila*, *Shala* and *Shaylah*.

### Shaylee, Shaylyn *see* Shea

### Shayne *see* Shane

### Shea *m. and f.*
This is the Irish surname Shea or *Shee* used as a
first name, most often in the USA. It comes from
an early-Irish first name Sé, meaning 'hawk-like'.
Rather than suggesting an aggressive person, it
concentrated on the beauty of the hawk and came
to have the sense 'fine, stately, goodly'. It is also

found as *Shay* and *Shaye*, and as a girl's name has developed the elaborations *Shaylee* and *Shaylyn*.

## Sheary *see* Séafraid

## Shee *see* Shea

## Sheedy *Síoda* m.

This unusual name, associated especially with the MacNamara family, may come from a word for 'silk'.

## Sheela, Sheelagh, Sheelah *see* Sheila

## Sheena, Sheenagh *see* Sine

## Sheila *Síle* f.

Síle is the Irish form of St *Cecilia*'s name. As well as Sheila, it has been anglicized in all sorts of spellings: *Shelagh*, *Sheelagh*, *Shilla*, *Selia*, *Shela*, *Shelia*, *Sheilah*, *Sheile*, *Shiela*, *Sheela*, *Sheelah* and *Shelegh*, to name a few. *Shahla* is probably another variant of the name. In the USA at the moment **Shayla** (and its variants) is a rather more popular form, although Sheila and its variants are also used. St Cecilia (also known as Cecily and Celia) was, according to her legend, a noble Roman lady – her name is a form of a well-attested Roman name, which came ultimately from the Latin word meaning 'blind' – who was martyred for her Christian faith in the third century. Her role as the patron saint of music seems to come from the story that, at her wedding, 'as the organs were playing Cecilia sung to the Lord, saying: may my heart remain unsullied, so that I be not confounded'. Cecilia was later re-adapted into Irish as *Sisile*.

**Shemus** *see* **Seamus**

**Shena** *see* **Sine**

**Sheridan** *m.*
This Irish surname, as borne by Irish playwright Richard Brinsley Sheridan (1751–1816), is used as a first name. The most famous current holder is probably the critic and writer Sheridan Morley (whose name is abbreviated to **Sherry**). The source of the surname is an Irish first name *Sirideán*, the meaning of which is not known.

**Sheron** *see* **Seathrún**

**Sherry** *see* **Sheridan**

**Shevaun** *see* **Siobhan**

**Shevon** *see* **Shavon**

**Shiela, Shilla** *see* **Sheila**

**Shivaun** *see* **Siobhan**

**Shivon, Shivonne, Shovon** *see* **Shavon**

**Sibéal** *f.*

This is the Irish form of *Isabel* or *Isobel*. Isabel itself is a medieval form of *Elizabeth*, which appears in Ireland as **Eilis**. *Sibby* is a pet form.

**Síle** *see* **Sheila**

**Simidh** *see* **Seamus**

**Sinan, Sinon** *see* **Senan**

**Síne** *f.*

Síne is an Irish form of *Jane* (see **Sinead** for further details), in its turn a feminine form of the name *John* (see **Sean**). Síne is better-known outside Ireland in the form *Sheena* (as in the singer Sheena Easton), originally a Scots–Gaelic anglicization of the name. The form *Sine* is used in the USA alongside Sheena, *Sheenagh* and *Shena*.

**Sinead** *Sinéad f.*

Sinead, like **Síne** and **Siobhan**, is an Irish form of the name *Jane*. In the middle ages *John* (see **Sean**) was one of the most popular names throughout Christendom, and a variety of ways were found in different countries of turning it into a girl's name. In English are the forms Jane, Janet and Joan, all from this root. In medieval French there were the forms Jeanne, Jehanne, and Jeanette. The first of these became Síne, the next Siobhan, while Jeanette became Sinead. All these connections seem to have been overlooked by those who translated Sinead into more familiar English names, for it took on a bewildering variety of shapes, only a few of them connected with the name's source: Susan, Judith, Judy, Johanna, Hannah, Susanna, Julia and the peculiar Jude and Nonie. Sinéad can also be found as *Sineaid*, while *Sinéidín* is a pet form. Sinead is very popular in Ireland at the moment, and has become well-known elsewhere through the actress Sinead Cusack and the singer Sinead O'Connor.

## Siobhan *Siobhán f.*

Siobhan is another Irish form of *Jane* (see **Sinead** for further details), and is usually regarded as the Irish for *Joan*. It has been very popular in Ireland and has spread to other English-speaking countries where, because of the difficulties Irish spelling presents to the uninitiated, it has developed an outlandish variety of forms. The commonest form in the USA is **Shavon**, and related variants have been listed under this heading. Another group of spellings are *Chavon*, *Chevonne* and *Chivonne*. The Irish playwright **Sean** O'Casey's daughter is the director *Shivaun* O'Casey, and the name can also be found as *Shevaun*. In Irish the name can also be found as *Siubhán* with pet forms *Siubháinín* or *Siobháinín*. This pet form is often thought of as the Irish for *Josephine* (but see also **Seosaimhín**). The standard spelling of the name has become familiar through the actress Siobhán McKenna. An earlier bearer was the daughter of Gerald, third Earl of Desmond (1359–98), or Gearóid Iarla. She was married to one Tadhg or **Tad** MacCarthy, who had enjoyed reputation of 'the most celebrated wine-bibber of his age'. As her father had been granted control of the wine trade in Ireland by the English crown, one is forced to wonder at her husband's motives for the marriage.

**Síoda** *see* **Sheedy**

**Siofraidh** *see* **Séafraid**

**Siomaidh, Síomaigh, Siomataigh** *see* **Seamus**

**Sionán** *see* **Senan**

**Siothrún** *m.*
This is yet another Irish adaptation of *Geoffrey*,

although the name is more likely to occur in the forms listed under **Séafraid** and **Seathrún**.

## Sirideán *see* **Sheridan**

## Sisile *see* **Sheila**

## Sitric *m*.

Sitric was used by Dublin's medieval Viking kings, most notably Sitric Silk-beard (for whom see under **Gormlaith**), and is still occasionally found. In the past it was well enough used to have been the source of the Irish surname MacKitterik or Kitterick, via the form Mac Shitric, 'son of Sitric'.

## Siubháinín, Siubhán *see* **Siobhan**

## Siúi *Sósaidh* f.

These are the Irish spellings of Sue and Susie, the pet forms of **Susan** (in Irish *Súsanna*). The name comes from the Hebrew for 'lily' and came into use from the story in the biblical *Apocrypha*, popular in the Middle Ages, of how the virtuous and clever Susannah, when being blackmailed by the lustful Elders to commit adultery, tricked them into revealing their own deceit. There is also a St Susanna, martyred in the third century for refusing to marry a relative of the great persecutor of Christians, the emperor Diocletian.

## Siún *f.*

Siún is occasionally found in Ireland as an adaptation of *Joan*. However, most Irish people, asked for the Irish for Joan, would suggest **Siobhan**.

## Sive *Sadhbh f.*

Thought to mean 'goodness' or 'sweetness', this was the name of the mother of **Ossian**. There are differing versions of her story, but one relates that on a hunting trip **Finn** Mac Cool came across a fawn that his hounds refused to attack. His sparing her must have broken a spell, for that night a beautiful woman came to him and told him that she was Sive, and has been turned into a fawn by the Dark Druid. She became his mistress but one day, while she was pregnant and Finn was away hunting, the Dark Druid found Sive again and turned her back into a deer. All Finn knew when he returned was that she had disappeared, but when he later found a child in the wood who had been raised by a deer, he knew it must be his son by Sive and named him Ossín, or 'little deer'. Sive has long been a popular name in Ireland, and was also anglicized as *Sabia* and *Sabine*, while the pet form *Saidhbhín* became *Sabena* or *Sabina*. All these are still used, although historically Sabina was also used to anglicize *Síle* (see **Sheila**). In origin, Sabine or Sabina is a Latin name meaning 'Sabine woman', the Sabines being a neighbouring tribe to the original Latins who founded Rome.

## Sivney *Suibhne m.*

Suibhne is most often anglicized as *Sweeney*, and is the source of the surname. However, the lasting infamy of Sweeney Todd, the late-eighteenth-century barber who supposedly murdered his clients and passed the bodies on to a nearby bakery to be baked into meat pies, has made it difficult to use Sweeney as a first name, and users are forced to turn to an alternative form for an anglicization. Suibhne Geilt (Mad Sweeny) is a famous character, part of whose story is told under **Ronan**. After St Ronan Finn had cursed him Sweeny went mad and took to the woods, sheltering in the trees and travelling Ireland as a wild bird-man. Mad Sweeny has played an important role in twentieth-century literature, appearing the poems of W. B. Yeats and T. S. Eliot, and featuring in **Flann** O'Brien's novel, *At Swim-Two-Birds* (1939).

## Slany *Sláine f.*

In use since the late Middle Ages, Slany comes

from the Irish word for 'health'. It can also be found in the Latin form Slanina, and has been exported to France in the forms *Slania* and *Slanie*.

## Somerled, Somhairle *see* Sorley

## Sorcha *f.*

Sorcha means 'bright, radiant', and is also used as an Irish equivalent of Sarah or Sally. It has been used increasingly in Ireland and is growing in popularity in Britain, its spread no doubt helped by the fame of the actress Sorcha Cusack.

## Sorley *Somhairle m.*

This is the Irish form of an Old Norse name Sumarlithr, meaning 'summer wanderer', the term for a Viking. The Vikings, for whom Ireland and the Scottish islands represented the warm south, would winter at home while the seas were rough and go raiding richer lands in the summer. The Scots turned the name into *Somerled* or *Summerlad*, while Somhairle is common to both forms of Gaelic. The form *Samhairle* is also found in Ireland. One famous holder of the name was Sorley Boy MacDonnell (1505–90). Of mixed Irish and Scots Highlander stock, his family were politically active on both sides of the Irish Sea. Large numbers of Highlanders settled in Antrim, and were regarded with suspicion by both Elizabeth I and **Shane** the Proud O'Neill, the greatest power in Ulster. Sorley Boy fought Shane and came off worse, but after Shane's death he fought the English, who were determined to expel the Scots from Ireland. After a life of mixed success and great hardship he submitted to the queen, was granted the right to hold his Irish lands in peace, and became one of the few great chieftains of that turbulent age to die quietly in their beds. The 'Boy' element of his name is a corruption of the Irish *buidhe*, 'yellow' and referred to his hair. A more recent holder of the name was Somhairle McCana (1901–75), a Belfast-born painter and designer.

### Sósaidh *see* Siúi

### Standish, Stanislaus *see* Aneslis

### Suibhne *see* Sivney

### Summerlad *see* Sorley

### Susan, Súsanna *see* Siúi

### Sweeney *see* Sivney

### Synan *see* Senan

# t

## Tad Tadhg m.

Tad is an anglicization, used especially in the USA, of the Irish name Tadgh, or 'poet'. It is also anglicized as *Teigue*, *Teague* and *Taig*, but the last two are also used as offensive terms for a Catholic by northern anti-Catholic bigots. The spellings *Tadgh* and *Tighe* have been recorded, although they are not standard Irish. *Tadleigh*, *Tadhgán* and *Taidhgín* are pet forms. In the past the name was translated Thaddeus, Theophilus and Theodosius, helping to keep these obscure Greek names alive, and *Thady* became a standard anglicization. Today *Timothy* is the commonest equivalent. In modern Irish Tadhg is used in set phrases as an alternative for 'man'; so, for example, 'Tadhg na sráide' is 'the man in the street'. The name occurs in mythology in the Munster nobleman Tadhg Mac Céin, whose attempts to win back his abducted wife took him on an Odyssean journey through strange lands.

## Talulla *Tuilelaith* f.

Talulla means 'lady of abundance', and is cropping up more frequently in birth announcements. It is most often spelt *Tallulah*, a form made famous by the outrageous film star Tallulah Bankhead (1903–68). It was not a stage name, but was inherited from her grandmother, and could have had two sources: either the Irish name, or the Tallulah Falls in Georgia, not far from her birthplace. (The falls got their name from a Native American word said to mean 'terrible'.) The Irish name is an old one and was borne by two saints, one an eighth-century abbess of Clonguffin, Co. Meath, and a second who was abbess of Kildare and died in 885.

## Tara *Teamhair* f.

Tara is the name of the great series of prehistoric remains dating from as early as 2000 BC, well before the arrival of the Gaelic peoples in Ireland. Around 500 BC the Gaels made it their royal centre, the seat of their high king and the centre of the religious activities that went with the kingship. Tara features prominently in the stories of early kings and heroes. In myth, it is supposed to have got its name from Tea, the wife of *Éireamhóin* who came with him from Spain to Ireland (see further under **Éibhear**). In Spain she had seen a rampart around a noblewoman's

241

grave, and once in Ireland asked her husband to give her the hill at what became Tara so she could build something similar. She was duly buried there, giving her name to the place. But in reality Tara seems simply to mean 'place commanding a fine prospect', or 'a crag'. The name has been used since the late-nineteenth century, but was rare until given heavy exposure outside Ireland. The book and film of *Gone With the Wind* (1939) brought it to a vast audience, and it was further boosted in the 1960s by a character in *The Avengers* TV series. Tara is nearly always used as a girl's name, but it has been used for boys, as in the case of Tara Guinness, whose early death in a motor accident inspired the Beatles song, *A Day in the Life*. It is well used across the English-speaking world, and is currently popular in Ireland and in the USA, where forms such as *Tarah*, *Tarra*, *Tarrah* and even *Tera* and *Terra* have been recorded.

**Taren, Tarin** *see* **Tyrone**

**Tarla, Tárlach, Tárnaigh** *see* **Turlough**

**Tarra, Tarrah** *see* **Tara**

**Taryn** *see* **Tyrone**

## Teabóid *m.*

Teabóid or **Tiobóid** is the Irish form of the Germanic name **Theobald**, made up of elements meaning 'people' and 'brave'. Although not much used now, Theobold has been a prominent name in Irish history. Theobald the Butler (d. c.1205) was the first royal butler of Ireland, a rank he was given when he accompanied Prince John of England to Ireland. His job became the family surname, and he was the founder of the Butler family (later Earls of Ormonde) who played such an important role in Irish history. The next five heads of his family were also Theobald. Theobold Burke, Viscount Mayo, was the son of the pirate Grace O'Malley (see **Grania**). He was also known as *Tibbot* of the Ships, as he was born at sea; indeed, his mother is said to have fought a battle immediately after his birth. The patriot Theobold Wolfe Tone (1763–98) co-founded the United Irishmen.

## Teafa *see* Teffia

## Teague *see* Tad

## Teamhair *see* Tara

## Teàrlach *see* Turlough

### Teffia *Teafa* f.

This unusual name is actually the old name of a district in Co. Longford, but in myth Teffia appears as the daughter of **Eochaidh** Aireamh. As his second name means 'the ploughman' and his story seems to be a distant memory of agricultural myths, it is not surprising to find the name of a piece of land incorporated into his family.

### Teigue *see* Tad

### Tel *see* Terence

### Tera, Terra *see* Tara

### Terence m.

Terence is not Irish, but an ancient Roman name, borne by the great playwright who lived in the second century BC. However, it was used so frequently to translate **Turlough** that it has become thought of as an Irish name. The writer Rudyard Kipling, for example, used Terence Mulvaney as the name of his Irish private soldier in the British army in India in the late nineteenth century. Language authorities nowadays translate Terence as *Traolach*. Terence is shortened to *Terry* and *Tel*, as in the case of Terry Wogan, the TV and radio presenter. Terence is still very common in

Ireland and is currently quite popular in the USA where it is most often spelt *Terrance* or *Terance*. It is also found as *Terrence*. *Terrell* (also the name of an American city), *Terris* and *Terron* may all be American developments of the name. Terry or *Terri* as a girl's name was originally a development of the name *Theresa* (see **Treasa**), but some users may no longer distinguish between masculine and feminine uses.

**Terran** *see* **Tyrone**

**Terrance, Terrell, Terrence, Terri, Terris, Terron, Terry** *see* **Terence**

**Teryn** *see* **Tyrone**

**Thady** *see* **Tad**

**Theobald** *see* **Teabóid**

**Theresa** *see* **Treasa**

**Thomas** *see* **Tomás**

**Tiarnach** *see* **Tierney**

**Tiarnán** *see* **Tiernan**

**Tibbot** *see* **Teabóid**

## Tiernan *Tiarnán* m.

Tiernan comes from *tigern*, 'lord, chief', and can also be found as *Tighearnán*. It was the name of Tiernan O'Ruairc (d. 1172), King of Brefni (Cavan and Leitrim). He and **Dermot** Mac Murrough, King of Leinster, were already political rivals when Tiernan's wife **Dervorgilla** (*Dearbhorgaill*, 'daughter of (the god) Forgall') ran off with the tall, handsome Dermot in 1151. The situation was made worse when Dermot tired of her and sent her back, but it was not until 1166 that Tiernan could take advantage of the political turmoil in Ireland and invade Dermot's kingdom. Dermot's brutal rule ensured that his kingdom rose in revolt, but his response, to seek new allies in England, was to lead to the arrival of the Norman invaders and the end of Irish independence.

## Tierney *Tiarnach* m. and f.

Tierney, like **Tiernan**, comes from the word *tigern*, 'lord'. The name is also spelt *Tighearnach*, while its old form, *Tigernach*, is used for St Tigernach of Clones (d. c.550). The illegitimate son of a ward of the king of Oriel, he was christened by St **Brigid** at Kildare. In his youth he was taken by pirates to Britain where he became a monk, later returning to Ireland and founding the monastery at Clones,

Co. Monaghan. Tierney is occasionally found in
the USA as a girl's name, in which case it is
probably taken directly from the surname (which
in turn comes from the first name). Its use may be
influenced by the actress Gene Tierney (1920–91).

## Tighe *see* Tad

## Tighearnach *see* Tierney

## Tighearnán *see* Tiernan

## Timothy *see* Tad

## Tiobóid *see* Teabóid

## Toal *see* Tuathal

## Toirdhealbhach *see* Turlough

## Toiréasa *see* Treasa

## Tomás *m.*

This is the Irish form of **Thomas**, the biblical name
meaning 'twin'. There is a pet form, *Tomáisín*.
In Irish folklore Tomás Mór ('Big Thomas') is the
founder of a clan of boorish, quarrelsome churls.
He is first found in an anonymous, early
seventeenth-century, satirical text called
*Pairlement Chloinne Tomáis* (The Parliament of Clan

Thomas), which formed a rich source of humorous invective and terms of abuse to be mined by later writers. There is some evidence that Tomás Mór may be meant to be a portrait of Black Thomas Butler (1532–1614), the tenth Earl of Ormonde, who was attacked for his active support of the English.

### Traoine *see* Catriona

### Traolach *see* Terence

### Treasa *f.*

Treasa or *Treise* is an old Irish name meaning 'strength' which has been adopted as an Irish equivalent of *Theresa*, more properly *Toiréasa*. It is used firstly in honour of the spiritual writer and mystic St Theresa of Ávila (1515–82) who founded the reformed Carmelite Order of nuns, and secondly of St Theresa of Lisieux (1873–97), 'the Little Flower', a Carmelite nun whose account of her spiritual journey before her early death has been enormously influential. Theresa is a very common name in Ireland.

### Trina *see* Catrina

### Triona *Tríona f.*

This is a short form of the name **Catriona**, which

is sometimes used as an independent name.
In the same way, *Trina* is used as a short form
from the variant *Catrina*.

## Cuathal *m.*

This name means 'leader of the people', and
has been anglicized as *Toal* and *Tully*. The High
King Tuathal Teachtmhar ('possessing wealth') is
supposed to have ruled all Ireland in the second
century AD. While he may have been a historical
figure, the stories told of him are mythical, and
there certainly were no high kings at this date. It
was said to be the dishonour done to his daughter
**Darina** which brought about the tax on Leinster
that caused great conflict between the province
and the high king for generations. There is a
pretty but rare girl's name, *Tuathla* or *Thuathlaith*,
meaning 'princess of the people' which, as it
shares the same root, could be used as a feminine
form of the name.

## Cuilelaith *see* Calulla

## Cully *see* Cuathal

## Curlough Craolach *m.*

Turlough or *Turloch* is an anglicization of a name

once thought of as coming from the name of the Norse Thunder god, Thor; but it is now believed to derive from an Irish word meaning 'instigator, abettor'. The old spelling of the name's Irish form, *Toirdhealbhach*, was used by the writer T. H. White in *The Once and Future King*. It is also found in the forms *Tárnaigh*, *Tárlach* and *Tarla*, and was translated **Charles**. The Scottish form *Teàrlach* was also used for Charles, and was used, for example, for the name of Bonnie Prince Charlie. Turlough was also anglicized as *Turley* and translated most often as **Terence** or *Terry*, and is the main source of these names in Ireland. Turlough was a common name among eleventh- and twelfth-century kings, including Turlough O'Brien, King of Munster and claimant of the high kingship, who died in 1086 at the then-great age of seventy-seven. His namesake fought the Norman invaders for his hereditary land of Thomond, Co. Clare, from 1276 to 1318, and was the subject of the laudatory *The Wars of Turlough*, written in Irish some fifty years later. The name was also used by several prominent members of the O'Connor family, including Turloch Donn ('the brown') O'Connor and Turloch Ruadh ('the red') O'Connor, who were rivals for the kingship of Connacht in the fourteenth century.

## Tyrone m.

Tyrone is the county name used as a first name. The place-name means 'Eoghan's land', being originally land occupied by those who claimed descent from **Eoghan** Mór (see that entry for more details). The name has been prominent in the theatrical world in the twentieth century in the persons of the English director Tyrone Guthrie (1900–71) and the American actor Tyrone Power (1913–58). The name was a family one: both had the same great-grandfather, the Waterford-born actor and playwright Tyrone Power (1797–1841). However, it has now spread and is not uncommon in the USA, where it is shortened to *Ty* and can also appear as *Tyron*. Tyrone Power and his wife, the actress Linda Christian, invented a development of his name for their daughter, whom they called *Taryn*. This name was taken up by others, and appears also in the forms *Taren*, *Tarin*, *Terran* and *Teryn*. The model *Tyra* Banks shows another feminine form of the name.

# U

**Uaine, Uainthne, Uaitne** *see* **Owny**

**Uilleac, Uilleag** *see* **Ulick**

## Uilliam *m.*
The Irish form of the Germanic name *William*, made up of elements meaning 'will, desire' and 'helmet, protection'. Although originally a short form, **Liam** is now a much more common form of the name.

## Uinseann *m.*
This name, meaning 'conquering', is the Irish form of *Vincent*, used in honour of St Vincent De Paul (c.1580–1660). He co-founded the Sisters of Charity, the first congregation of 'unenclosed' women devoted to the care of the poor and sick. He was also active in missionary work, and Ireland, where the Catholic faith was then

persecuted, was one of the countries to which he sent missionaries. The name is also found as *Uinsionn*.

## Ulick *Uilleag* m.

This popular name is generally thought of as from a pet form of *Uilliam*, although one theory makes it a borrowing from the Norse. Also spelt *Uilleac* in Irish, it has been anglicized as *Ulysses*, adding a further dimension to James Joyce's novel of that name. There is a rare feminine form, *Ulicia*.

## Ultan *Ultán* m.

Ultan means 'an Ulsterman' and was the name of eighteen Irish saints. One of these, who died in 686, was one of three saintly brothers who worked in France. His cult spread through France and into Belgium. Another, Ultan of Ardbraccan (d. 657), was a scholar who wrote a life of St **Brigid**, had a reputation for feeding and clothing poor students, and is the patron saint of children.

## Ulysses *see* Ulick

## Una *Úna* f.

This popular name is also found nowadays anglicized as *Oonagh* or *Oona*. **Juno** is also said to be a form, but there is little evidence to support this. A well known song, *Úna Bhán*, ('Fair Una'), tells of the tragic love between Úna Mac Dermott and Tomás Láidir Costello. It is generally said that when Edmund Spenser chose the name Una for the heroine of *The Faerie Queene* he was thinking not of the Irish name, but of the Latin sense of the word 'one' (hence the fact that the Irish Una is sometimes translated *Unity*). However, Spenser did spend time in Ireland, and various names he used in his epic poem can be traced to Irish sources: for example, *Artegal* (see under **Ardal**), and *Alma* (see *Almha* under **Alva**); while even his villainess Duessa could be linked to the name *Duibheasa*, 'dark lad of the waterfall', so that there is no reason why his names should not carried had both Irish and Latin senses.

# ꝺ-ɣ

## Vanessa *f.*

Jonathan Swift (1667–1745), the Dublin-born
satirist, poet and dean of St Patrick's Cathedral,
had a close but undefined relationship with a
woman called Esther Vanhomrigh whom he met
on a visit to London. Probably against his wishes,
she insisted on following him to Dublin, where
he wrote the poem *Cadenus and Vanessa* as
both a tribute to her and as a manoeuvre of
disengagement. The first name of the title is an
anagram of *decanus*, the Latin for 'dean', i.e.
Swift; while Vanessa, a partial anagram of her
name but sufficiently obscure not to bring shame
on her, was invented for this poem. Vanessa does
not seem to have entered the general stock of
names until the last hundred years or so.

## Vergil *see* **Fergal**

**Verity** *see* **Fírinne**

**Vigean** *see* **Fechin**

**Vincent** *see* **Uinseann**

**Virgil** *see* **Fergal**

**Vivian** *see* **Bevin**

**Webby** *see* **Gobnet**

**William** *see* **Liam, Uilliam**

**Yseult** *see* **Iseult**

# Appendix 1:
# English–Irish names

This list has two types of entry. The first, using '=', as in 'Alan = Ailín', shows the Irish form of an English name. The second, with the term 'used for', as in 'Albert used for Ailbe', shows the English name used to translate an Irish one. These translations from the Irish are also used in reverse today, when a name such as Albert, with no direct Irish form, may be translated in turn into Irish as Ailbe.

| | |
|---|---|
| **A**aron | = Árón |
| Abbie | = Abaigh, used for Gobnait (**Gobnet**) |
| Abigail | = Abaigeal, used for Gobnait (**Gobnet**) |
| Abraham | = Ábraham |
| Adam | = Ádhamh, Ádam |
| Adrian | = Aidrian |
| Aeneas | used for Aonghus (**Aengus**), Éigneachán (**Eneas**) |
| Agatha | = Agata, used for Mór |
| Agnes | = Aignéis, used for Úna |
| Alan | = Ailín |
| Alban | = Albán |
| Albert | used for Ailbe (**Alby**) |
| Alexander, Alaistair | = Alsander, Alastar |
| Alexandra | = Alastríona |

# English–Irish names

| | |
|---|---|
| Alfred | = Ailfrid |
| Alice | = Ailís, used for Aislinn |
| Alicia | = Ailíse |
| Alison | = Allsún |
| Aloysius | = Alaois, Alabhaois, used for Lughaidh |
| Amelia | = Aimilíona |
| Anastasia | = Annstás |
| Andrew | = Aindréas, Aindriú, Aindrias |
| Angela | = Aingeal |
| Anna, Anne | = Ánna, used for Áine, Eithne |
| Annabel(la) | = Annábla |
| Annie | used for Eithne |
| Anthony | = Antoin, Antóin, Antain(e), used for Uaithne (**Owny**) |
| Archibald | used for Giolla Easpie (**Gillespie**) |
| Arnold | used for Ardgal (**Ardal**) |
| Arthur | = Artúr, used for Art |
| Augustine | = Ághaistín, Aibhistín, Águistín, Ághuistín |
| Austin | = Oistín |
| **B**arbara | = Bairbre, Báirbre; pet form, Baibín, used for Gormlaith |
| Barnaby | = Barnaib, used for Brian |
| Bartholomew | = Bairtlméad, also used for Parthalán |
| Basil | used for Breasal (**Brassal**) |
| Benedict | used for Maolbheannachta |
| Bernard | = Bearnárd, used for Brian |
| Bertie | used for Ailbe |
| Blanche | used for Blinne |
| **C**atherine | = Caitrín, Caitlín, etc. |
| Cecily | = Síle (**Sheila**), Sisile |

| | |
|---|---|
| Charles | = Séarlas, Carlus, also used for Calbhach (**Calvagh**), Cathair (**Cahir**), Cathal (**Cahal**), Cearbhall, Cormac, Somhairle (**Sorley**), Traolach (**Turlough**) |
| Charlotte | = Séarlait, Charlot |
| Christian | used for Giolla Chríst (**Gillespie**) |
| Christina | = Crístíona |
| Christine | = Cristín |
| Christopher | = Críostóir |
| Clare | = Clár, Clare |
| Colin | = Coilín, Coileán |
| Constantine | used for Conn |
| Cornelius, Corney | used for Conchobhar (**Conor**) |
| Cyril | = Ciorail, Coireall |
| **Daisy** | used for Nóra |
| Daniel | used for Domhnall (**Donal**) |
| Darby | used for Diarmit (**Dermot**) |
| David | = Dáibhí, Daibhead |
| Debby, Deborah | used for Gobnait (**Gobnet**) |
| Denis | used for Donagh |
| Dolly | used for Doireann (**Dorean**) |
| Dominic | = Damhnaic, Damhlaic, Doiminic |
| Dora | used for Gobnait (**Gobnet**) |
| Dorothy | used for Devorgilla (**Tiernan**), Doireann (**Dorean**) |
| Dudley | used for Dara and Dubhaltach (**Duald**) |
| **Edmund** | = Éamon(n) |
| Edna | = Eithne |
| Edward | = Éadbhárd, used for Éamon(n) |
| Edwina | = Éadaoin |

259

| | |
|---|---|
| Eleanor | = Eileanóra, Eileanóir, Ailionóra |
| Elizabeth | = Eilís |
| Emily | = Eimíle |
| Ernest | used for Ernan |
| Esther | = Eistir, used for Aislinn |
| Eugene | used for Aodh, Eoghan |
| Eustace | = Iústás |
| Eva | = Éabha, used for Aoife |
| **Fa**nny | = Próinséas, used for Fainche |
| Felix | used for Feidhlim (**Phelim**) |
| Ferdinand, Ferdie | used for Feardhach (**Farry**), Fearadorcha (**Fardoragh**), Fearghus (**Fergus**) |
| Festus | used for Fachtna (**Fachnan**), Feichín (**Fechin**), Fiacha (**Fiach**) |
| Flora | used for Bláth (**Bláthnait**), Fionnuala (**Finola**) |
| Florence (*f*) | used for Bláthnait |
| Frances | = Proinséas |
| Francis | = Proinsias |
| Frank | = Frainc |
| Frederick | used for Feardhach (**Farry**), Feardorcha (**Fardoragh**) |
| **Ga**briel | = Gabriel, Gaibrial |
| Gareth | = Gairiad |
| Geoffrey | = Siothrún, Seathrún, Sheary |
| George | = Seoirse |
| Gerald | = Gearóid |
| Gerard | = Gearárd |
| Gertrude, Gertie | used for Gráinne (**Grania**) |

| | |
|---|---|
| Gilbert | = Gilibeirt, used for Giolla Bhríde (**Gillespie**) |
| Godfrey | = Gofraidh, Gothfraidh, Gofraí |
| Gordon | = Gordan |
| Grace | used for Gráinne (**Grania**) |
| Graham | = Gréachán |
| Gregory | = Gréagóir, Greagoir |
| Grisselda | used for Gráinne (**Grania**) |
| **H**annah | used for Áine, Onóra (**Honor**), Siobhán |
| Harold | = Aralt |
| Harry | used for Éibhear |
| Hector | used for Eachann |
| Helen, Helena | = Léan, Léana |
| Henry | = Anraí, Einrí, Annraoi, Han(n)raoi |
| Herbert | = Hoireabard |
| Hilary | = Hioláir |
| Hilda | = Hilde |
| Hubert | = Hoibeard |
| Hugh, Hughie | used for Aodh, Eoghan, Cúmhái (**Quintin**) |
| Humphrey | used for Amhlaoibh (**Auliffe**) |
| **I**rving | used for Éireamhóin (**Éibhear**) |
| Isaac | = Íosac |
| Isabel | = Isibéal, Sibéal |
| Ivor | = Íomhar, used for Éibhear |
| **J**ames | = Séamas, etc. |
| Jamie | = Séimí |
| Jane | = Síne |
| Janet | = Sinéad |

| | |
|---|---|
| Jasper | = Geaspar |
| Jeremiah, Jerome | used for Diarmait (**Dermot**) |
| Jeremy | used for Diarmait (**Dermot**) |
| Joan | = Siobhán |
| John | = Eoin, Séan, etc., used for Eoghan |
| Jonathan | = Seonac, Ionatán |
| Joseph | = Seosamh, Iósep(h) |
| Josephine | = Seosaimhín |
| Judith | used for Síle (**Sheila**), Siobhan |
| Judy | used for Síle (**Sheila**), Siobhán |
| Julia | = Iúile, used for Síle (**Sheila**), Siobhán |
| **K**ate | = Cáit |
| Kenneth, Kenny | used for Coinneach (**Canice**) |
| **L**aurence | = Labhrás, used for Lorcán |
| Lazarus | used for Lasairian (**Laserian**) |
| Leo | = Léon |
| Lily | = Líle |
| Louis, Lewis | used for Laoiseach (**Lysagh**), Lughaidh |
| Louise | = Labhaoise |
| Lucius | used for Lachtna, Laoighseach (**Lysagh**) |
| Luke | = Lúcás |
| **M**abel | = Máible, used for Meadhbh (**Maeve**) |
| Madeleine | = Madailéin |
| Madge | used for Muirinn (**Muireann**) |
| Malcolm | = Maolcholuim |
| Marcel | = Mairsile |
| Marcella | = Mairsile |
| Margaret | = Mairéad |
| Marion | used for Muirinn (**Muireann**) |
| Marjory | used for Meadhbh (**Maeve**) |

| | |
|---|---|
| Mark | = Marcas, Marcus |
| Martha | = Marta, used for Mór |
| Martin | = Máirtín, Mártan, Mártain |
| Mary | = Máire, Moira, Maura, Máirin, etc., used for Mór |
| Matilda | = Maitilde |
| Matthew | = Maitú, Matha, used for Mathúin (**Mahon**) |
| Matthias | = Maitias, Maithias |
| Maud | = Máda, used for Meadhbh (**Maeve**) |
| Maurice | = Muiris, used for Muiríos (**Muiris**) |
| Melissa | used for Maoilísa |
| Michael | = Míchaél, Micheál |
| Monica | = Moncha |
| Morgan | used for Murchadh (**Murrough**) |
| Mortimer | used for Muireartach (**Murtagh**), Murchadh (**Murrough**) |
| Moses | = Maois, Maoise, used for Manus |
| **N**ancy | = Nainsí |
| Nell | = Neile |
| Nicholas | = Nioclás, Nicol, used for Aonghus (**Aengus**), Niall |
| Norman | = Normán |
| **O**live | used for Ailbhe (**Alby**) |
| Oliver | = Oilibhéar |
| Owen | used for Eoghan, Eoin |
| **P**atricia | = Pádraigín |
| Patrick | = Pádraig |
| Paul | = Pól |
| Pauline | = Póilín |

| | |
|---|---|
| Penelope, Penny | used for Fionnuala (**Finola**), Nuala |
| Peter | = Feoras , Peadar, Piaras |
| Philip | = Pilib, used for Feidhlim (**Phelim**) |
| Piers | = Feoras, Piaras |
| Polly | = Paili |
| **R**achel | = Ráichéal |
| Ralph | = Rádhulbh |
| Randolph | = Rannulbh |
| Raymond | = Réamann, Redmond |
| Regina | used for Raghnailt, Ríona |
| Richard | = Ristéard, Riocard |
| Robert | = Roibéard |
| Roland | = Rólann |
| Rolf | = Rodhulbh |
| Rose | = Róis |
| Ruth | = Rut |
| **S**ally | used for Sadhbh (**Sive**), Sorcha |
| Samuel | used for Somhairle (**Sorley**) |
| Sarah | used for Saraid, Sadhbh (**Sive**), Sorcha |
| Simon | = Síomón, used for Suibhne (**Sivney**) |
| Sophie, Sophia | used for Sadhbh (**Sive**) |
| Stacey | = Stéise |
| Stanislaus | used for Ainéislis (**Aneslis**) |
| Stephen | = Stiofán, Stiana |
| Susan | = Súsanna, used for Siobhán |
| Susanna | used for Siobhán |
| **Th**addeus, Thady | used for Tadhg (**Tad**) |
| Theobald | = Tiobóid |
| Theresa | = Toiréasa |
| Thomas | = Tomás |

| | |
|---|---|
| Tim | used for Tadhg (**Tad**) |
| Toby | = Tóibí, used for Tadhg (**Tad**) |
| **U**lysses | used for Uilleag (**Ulick**) |
| Unity | used for Úna |
| **V**alentine | = Bhailintín |
| Victor | used for Buadhach (**Buagh**) |
| Vincent | = Uinsean |
| Virgil, Vergil | = Firgil, used for Fearghal (**Fergal**) |
| Vivian (*f*) | used for Béibhinn (**Bevin**) |
| **W**alter | = Ualtar, Uaitár |
| William | = Uilliam, Liam |
| Winifred | used for Úna |

# Appendix 2:
# Pronunciation guide

This list shows general pronunciations for Irish names in the A–Z which would be difficult for a non-Irish speaker to work out; note that regional accents can produce slightly different pronunciations from those given here. Capitals denote the syllable in a name which should be stressed.

| | | | |
|---|---|---|---|
| Ádhamh | AU'v | Ailis | Al-ice |
| Adamnan | Eye-oo-naun | Ailish | Ile-eesh |
| Adomnan | Ad-oo-naun | Aindrias | An-DREEAS |
| Aed | Ey | Aindriú | Androo |
| Aedan | Ey-dan | Áine | Oyn-nyeh |
| Aeneas | Ey-NEY-as | Ainéislis | An-EYSH-lish |
| Aengus | Eyn-gus | Ainmire | En-MIRR-eh |
| Ághaistín | EY-ash-teen | Airtín | Art-een |
| Aghna | EY-na | Aisling | Ash-ling |
| Aibhílín | Ov-leen | Aislinn | Ash-ling |
| Aibhistín | Ov-is-teen | Alabhaois | Al--ov-eesh |
| Aibhne | Ov-neh | Alaois | Al-eesh |
| Aignéis | Ag-NEYSH | Alastriona | Al-as-TRI-ona |
| Ailbe | Al-BEH | Alayna | Al-EY-na |
| Ailbhe | Al-VEH | Almha | Al-va |
| Aileen | Oil-een | Almu | AL-mas |
| Ailine | Oil-in-nyeh | Aloisia | Al-OY-sa |
| Ailís | Al-eesh | Aloysius | Alo-ish-us |

# Pronunciation guide

| | |
|---|---|
| Amhalgaidh | Owl-ghee |
| Amhlaoibh | Owl-lee |
| Annábla | On-AUB-la |
| Anvirre | AN-virr-eh |
| Aodán | Ey-daun |
| Aodh | Ey |
| Aodhach | Ey-uk |
| Aodhagán | Ey-gan |
| Aodhaigh | Ey-ee |
| Aodhamair | Ey-mir |
| Aodhan | Ey-gaun |
| Aodhfin | Ey-fin |
| Aodhfionn | Ey-fyunn |
| Aodhgan | Ey-gan |
| Aodhnait | Ey-nit |
| Aogán | Ey-gan |
| Aoibheann | Ee-van |
| Aoibhinn | Ee-vin |
| Aoife | EE-feh |
| Aonghas | Ey-nus |
| Ardgal | Argle |
| Ardghal | Argle |
| Artagán | Art-a-gaun |
| Artán | Art-aun |
| Artin | Art-een |
| Artúr | Ar-THOOR |
| Ashlin | Ash-ling |
| Ataigh | Att-ee |
| Athracht | Ah-hroct |
| Attracta | Att-RACT-a |

| | |
|---|---|
| Awnan | EYE-oo-naun |
| **B**accán | Bok-KAUN |
| Baibín | Bab-een |
| Báirbre | Bar-breh |
| Bairfhionn | BEER-inn |
| Bairre | BARR-eh |
| Bairrionn | BAR-inn |
| Banbha | BAN-vah |
| Banbhan | Ban-van |
| Banbhnait | Bonv-nit |
| Barnaby | BAR-na-bee |
| Barra | Borr-ah |
| Beag | Byug |
| Beagóg | Byug-ohg |
| Bean | Ban |
| Bean Mhí | Ban-vee |
| Bean Mhumhan | Ban-VOO-an |
| Beanón | Ban-ohn |
| Bearach | Bar-ak |
| Bearchán | Bar-u-kaun |
| Beartlaidh | BART-lee |
| Beatha | Ba-ha |
| Beathag | Ba-hag |
| Bébhinn | Bay-ving |
| Bec | Bek |
| Becan | Bek-aun |
| Bedelia | Be-DEEL-yah |
| Béibhinn | Bay-ving |
| Beineán | Ben-AUN |

267

# Pronunciation guide

| | | | |
|---|---|---|---|
| Beineón | Ben-ohn | Briartach | Bree-ar-thuk |
| Bethoc | Beh-hok | Bríd | Breed |
| Bidelia | Bi-DEEL-ia | Brídín | Breed-een |
| Bineán | Bin-AUN | Brieanna | Bree-na |
| Bláithín | Blaw-heen | Brighid | Breed |
| Blánaid | Blaw-nid | Brigid | BRIJ-id |
| Bláth | Blaw | Brigida | BRIJ-id-ah |
| Bláthnaid | Blaw-nid | Broc(k) | Bruk |
| Bláthnait | Blaw-nit | Brona | Broh-na |
| Bline | BLIH-ne | Brónach | Broh-nok |
| Blinne | BLIN-neh | Bronagh | Broh-nok |
| Bran | Bron | Brone | Brohn |
| Branagán | Bran-agaun | Bua(dha)ch | BOO-ak |
| Branán | Bran-aun | Buagh | BOO-ak |
| Brandan | Bran-dawn | | |
| Brandon | Bran-dun | Cabhán | Ka-VAUN |
| Brandubh | Bran-duav | Cadhan | KEYE-an |
| Braon | Brain | Cadla | KEYE-la |
| Braonán | Brain-aun | Caelainn | Kay-ling |
| Brasil | Brass-il | Cahal | Coh-ul |
| Breana | Brey-na | Cahir | Care |
| Bréanainn | Breyn-oin | Cainnech | Can-ek |
| Breandán(n) | BRAN-daun | Cairbre | Carb-reh |
| Breann | Bran | Cairenn | COR-ean |
| Breanna | Brey-na | Caisel | Cash-el |
| Breasal | Brass-ul | Caisín | Cash-een |
| Breaslán | Brass-laun | Caislín | Cash-leen |
| Breda | Bree-da | Caít | Koit |
| Breege | Breej | Caitilín | Koit-leen |
| Breonna | Bryoh-na | Caitlin | Kat-leen |

| | | | |
|---|---|---|---|
| Caitrín | Kot-reen | Catriona | Kat-REE-na |
| Caitríona | Kot-REE-on-a | Cavan | CAV-an |
| Calbhach | Kol-vok | Céadach | KAID-uk |
| Callaghan | KALL-a-han | Ceallach | KAL-uk |
| Canair | CON-ir | Ceallachán | KAL-uk-aun |
| Canice | Kan-is | Ceallagh | KAL-uk |
| Cansaidín | KON-sad-een | Cearbhall | Kar-ool |
| Caoilfhionn | KAIL-in | Cearúl(l) | Kar-ool |
| Caoilinn | KAIL-in | Chavon | Sha-VON |
| Caoilte | KWEEL-teh | Chevonne | Sheh-VON |
| Caoimhe | KEEV-eh | Chivonne | Shi-VON |
| Caoimhín | KEEV-een | Cian | KEE-an |
| Caoinleán | KEEN-laun | Cianán | KEE-an-aun |
| Caolán | KAIL-aun | Ciannait | KEE-an-nit |
| Caomhán | KAVE-aun | Ciar | KEER |
| Carey | Kare-ee | Ciara | KEER-a |
| Carraig | Korr-ig | Ciarán | KEER-aun |
| Carthagh | KOR-huk | Ciaran | KEER-aun |
| Carthach | KOR-huk | Ciarnait | KEER-nit |
| Carthage | KAR-thaj | Cleona | KLEE-na |
| Carthy | KAR-thee | Clídna | KLEE-na |
| Casey | KAY-see | Clíodhna | KLEE-oh-na |
| Cassán | KOSS-aun | Cliona | KLEE-na |
| Cathair | Koh-ir | Clodagh | KLOH-da |
| Cathal | Koh-hal | Cnochúr | KRUH-oor |
| Cathán | Koh-aun | Cóilín | KOHL-een |
| Cathaoir | Koh-eer | Coinneach | Kinnock |
| Cathasach | KOH-a-sok | Coll | Kull |
| Catheld | CAT-held | Colla | KULL-ah |
| Catrina | Kat-REE-na | Colleen | KOLL-een |

# Pronunciation guide

| | | | |
|---|---|---|---|
| Colma | KUL-mah | Cuán | KOO-aun |
| Colman | KUL-man | Cúchulainn | KOO-KULL-in |
| Colmán | KUL-maun | Cuimín | Kum-EEN |
| Coman | KOH-man | Cúmhái | KOO-voy |
| Comán | Ku-MAUN | Cú Mhaighe | KOO-voy |
| Comgall | KO-gal | Cumin | Kum-EEN |
| Comgan | KO-gan | Cummian | Kum-EEN |
| Comghán | KO-gan | | |
| Comhghall | KOH-gul | **D**abacc | DAV-ok |
| Comnait | KOH-nit | Dabag | DAV-ok |
| Comyn | KOM-in | Dabhag | DAV-ok |
| Conaire | KONN-er-eh | Dag(h)da | DIE-da |
| Conan | KOH-nan | Daibhead | DOY-vade |
| Conán | Kuh-NAUN | Daibhéid | DOY-vade |
| Conary | KONN-er-ee | Dáibhí | DOV-ee |
| Conchobarre | KRUH-oor | Daimhín | DAU-veen |
| Conchobhar | KRUH-oor | Dáire | DAU-reh |
| Connlao(dh) | KON-lee | Dáiríne | DAU-rin-ne |
| Connlaoi | KON-lee | Dairinn | DAU-rinn |
| Consaidín | KON-sa-deen | Dáithí | DAU-hee |
| Cormac | Kur-muk | Dálach | DAUL-uk |
| Corry | KORR-ee | Dallán | DALL-aun |
| Cory | KOHR-ee | Damhán | DOW-an |
| Crevan | KREE-van | Damhnait | DOW-nit |
| Criomhthann | KRIFF-in | Damhnat | DOW-nat |
| Criostal | Kristal | Dara | DARR-eh |
| Críostóir | Kree-us-TOR | Darach | DARR-eh |
| Crónán | Kroh-NAUN | Daragh | DARR-eh |
| Cronin | KROH-nin | Darerca | Da-RERK-ah |
| Cuan | KOO-an | Darina | Darr-EEN-ah |

| | | | |
|---|---|---|---|
| Darragh | DARR-eh | Donaghy | DON-a-hee |
| Deaglán | DEG-laun | Dónal | DOH-nul |
| Deamán | Dya-MAUN | Donall | DOH-nul |
| Dearbhail | DER-val | Donavan | DUN-a-van |
| Dearbhaile | DERV-la | Donegal | Dun-ee-GAUL |
| Dearbhla | DERV-la | Donie | DOH-nee |
| Dearbhorgaill | Der-vor-ghil | Donn | DOWN |
| Deasún | Dass-OON | Donnabhán | DUNN-a-vaun |
| Deidra | DEY-ra | Donnagán | DUNN-a-gaun |
| Deidr(i)e | DEY-ra | Donncha | DUNN-ak-ah |
| Deirbhile | DERV-leh | Donnchadh | DUNN-ak-a |
| Deirdre | DAIRD-reh | Dono(u)gh | DUNN-ah |
| Demitrius | De-MEET-ree-us | Doran | DOH-ran |
| Deoradhán | DYORE-a-han | Duald | DOO-ald |
| Derdriu | DERR-droo | Dualtach | DOO-al-thok |
| Derinn | DER-ing | Dualtagh | DOO-al-thok |
| Dervila | DER-vil-ah | Dubhaltach | DOO-al-tok |
| Dervorgilla | Der-vor-GHILL-ah | Dubhán | DOO-an |
| Desmumhnach | Des-MOON-uk | Dubhdara | DOO-dara |
| Diarmad | DEE-ar-mud | Dubhghall | DOO-al |
| Diarmaid | DEER-mid | Dúghail | DOO-al |
| Diarmait | DEER-mit | Duibheasa | DIV-i-sah |
| Diarmid | DEER-mid | Dúnlaith | DOON-lee |
| Diarmod | DEER-mod | | |
| Diarmuid | DEER-mud | | |
| Dierdra | DEER-dra | **Ea** | Ee-AH |
| Dierdrie | DEER-dree | Eacha | AK-a |
| Doireann | DUR-an | Eachann | AK-an |
| Domhnall | DOH-null | Eachdha | AK-ya |
| Donagh | DUN-ah | Eachdhonn | AK-un |
| | | Eachna | Ak-na |

## Pronunciation guide

| | | | |
|---|---|---|---|
| Éadaoin | Ade-een | Eireamhón | ER-ev-one |
| Ealga | Al-ga | Eireen | EYE-reen |
| Eamhair | AV-ir | Eirnín | ER-neen |
| Eamoinn | EY-mun | Eithne | ETH-neh |
| Eamon | EY-mun | Emer | EE-mir |
| Éanán | EY-naun | Emir | EE-mir |
| Éanna | EY-na | Emmet | EMM-et |
| Earc | Ark | Ena | EE-na |
| Earnán | AR-naun | Enan | EE-nan |
| Eavan | EV-in | Énán | EE-nane |
| Eavnat | EV-nat | Enat | Ey-nit |
| Edan | Ey-dan | Eneas | Ey-NEY-as |
| Eenis | Ey-NEY-as | Éneas | Ey-NEY-as |
| Egan | EE-gan | Enid | EE-nid |
| Éibhear | Ey-vir | Enos | EE-nos |
| Éibhleann | AVE-lan | Eny | EEN-ay |
| Eibhlín | EYE-leen | Enya | ENN-ya |
| Éigneach | EYG-nuk | Eoan | OH-an |
| Éigneachán | EYG-nuk-aun | Eochaí | YO-kee |
| Eileanóir | El-an-OHR | Eochaidh | YO-ee |
| Eiléanór | El-an-OHR | Eocho | YO-ko |
| Eileen | EYE-leen | Eoghan | OH-an |
| Eilíonóra | EYE-lee | Eoin | OH-in |
| Eilis | EYE-loosh | Erevan | ER-e-van |
| Eilís | EYE-leesh | Erin | EY-rin |
| Éimhear | EY-vir | Erina | Er-EEN-a |
| Éimhín | EY-veen | Ernan | Er-NAUN |
| Einín | EY-neen | Etain | Et-OIN |
| Éire | Ey-reh | Ethenia | Eh-THEEN-ee-a |
| Éireamhóin | ER-ev-one | Eugene | YOO-jeen |

| | | | |
|---|---|---|---|
| Eunan | YOO-nan | Feidhelm | FY-elm |
| Eva | EE-va | Feidhlim | FEY-lim |
| Evaline | EH-val-een | Feidhlimidh | FEY-lim-ee |
| Eveny | EEV-nee | Felan | FEE-lan |
| Ever | EE-vir | Felim | FEY-lim |
| Evin | EV-in | Felimid | FEY-lim-ee |
| | | Felimidh | FEY-lim-ee |
| Fachanan | FOK-nan | Felimy | FEY-lim-ee |
| Fachnan | FOK-nan | Fenella | Fe-NELL-ah |
| Fachtna | FOKT-na | Fenelly | FEN-ell-ee |
| Faenche | FAIN-ke | Feoras | FYOAR-ass |
| Fainche | FINE-ke | Fergal | FER-gal |
| Fainne | FAUN-ye | Fergus | FER-gus |
| Fania | FAUN-ye | Fiach | FEE-uk |
| Faolán | FWAY-laun | Fiacha | FEE-uk-ah |
| Fardoragh | Far-DOR-ah | Fiachra | FEE-uk-rah |
| Farquhar | FAR-har | Fiacre | FEE-uk-ur |
| Faughnan | FOK-nan | Fiadhnait | FEE-nit |
| Feagh | FEE-uk | Fiagh | FEE-uk |
| Fearadhach | Far-EY-ak | Fianait | FEE-nit |
| Fearchar | Fak-kur | Fidelma | Fi-DEL-ma |
| Feardorcha | Far-DHURR-ka | Fingal | FINN-gaul |
| Feargal | FAR-gal | Finghin | FIN-een |
| Fearghal | Farrell | Fíngin | FIN-een |
| Fearghus | FAR-us | Fínín | FEE-neen |
| Feary | FEE-ree | Finbarr | FINN-bar |
| Fechin | Feh-HEEN | Finnén | Fin-EYN |
| Fedelma | Fe-DEL-ma | Finnian | FINN-yan |
| Fehin | Feh-HEEN | Finola | Fi-NOH-lah |
| Feichín | Feh-HEEN | Fintan | FIN-tan |

# Pronunciation guide

| | | | |
|---|---|---|---|
| Fíona | FEE-onah | Gilchrist | Ghil-KREEST |
| Fiona | Fee-OH-nah | Gillespie | Ghil-ESS-pee |
| Fíonán | Fyun-AUN | Gilpatrick | Ghil-PAT-rick |
| Fionan | Fyun-AN | Giolla Bhríde | GHIL-la VREE-dah |
| Fionn | FYUNN | Giolla Chríst | GHIL-la KREE-ust |
| Fionnbhar | FYUN-var | Giolla Easpie | GHIL-la ASS-pee |
| Fionnbhárr | FYUN-var | Giolla Pádraig | GHIL-la PAUT-rik |
| Fionbharra | FYUN-vorrah | Giorárd | Gheer-AURD |
| Fionnghuala | Fyuh-NOO-lah | Gobinet | GUB-net |
| Fionntán | FYUN-taun | Gobnait | GUB-net |
| Fionnuala | Fyuh-NOO-lah | Gobnat | GUB-net |
| Fiontan | FYUN-tan | Gobnet | GUB-net |
| Firdorcha | Fir-DUR-ka | Gormflath | GURRM-leh |
| Fírinne | FEER-in-yeh | Gorm(fh)la(i)th | GURRM-leh |
| Fítheal | FIH-al | Grainne | GRAU-nyah |
| Flaithrí | FLAH-ree | Gráinne | GRAU-nyah |
| Flann | Flan | Grania | GRAU-nyah |
| Flannan | FLAN-an | Granina | Gre-NEEN-eh |
| Flannán | Flan-AUN | Granna | GRAU-nah |
| Flannchadh | FLAN-ka | Granya | GRAN-yah |
| | | | |
| **G**arbhán | GAR-vaun | **H**anora | Han-OH-rah |
| Garret(t) | GAR-ett | Hierlath | EE-AR-lah |
| Gearalt | GAR-alt | Honora | On-OH-rah |
| Gearárd | GAR-aurd | | |
| Gearóid | GAR-oh-id | **I**agan | EE-gan |
| Gearóidín | GAR-oh-deen | Iarfhlaith | EE-AR-lah |
| Gene | JEEN | Iarlaith | EE-AR-lah |
| Gerrit | GHER-it | Íd | Eed |
| Gilbride | Ghil-BRIDE | Íde | EED-eh |

| | | | |
|---|---|---|---|
| Idnat | EN-id | Lachtna | LOKT-nah |
| Ilene | EYE-leen | Lachtnán | LOKT-nan |
| Ina | EYE-nah | Laisren | LAIS-ren |
| Ineenduv | In-EEN-dhuv | Laisrián | Lash-RAUN |
| Iobhar | EE-ver | Laoighseach | LEE-shah |
| Iodhnait | EE-nat | Laoiseach | LEE-shah |
| Íonait | EE-nat | Lasair | LOH-sir |
| Iósep | YO-sep | Lasairian | Loh-SIRR-yan |
| Ióseph | YO-sef | Lasairíona | LOH-ser-EE-on-ah |
| Irial | IRR-yal | Laserian | La-SER-ee-an |
| Iseult | EE-sult | Lasrina | Lo-SREEN-ah |
| Isleen | EYE-leen | Lassar | LOSS-as |
| Ita | EE-ta | Lassarina | Loh-serr-EEN-ah |
| Ivar | EYE-var | Laughlin | LOK-lan |
| | | Leachlainn | LOK-lan |
| Jacinta | Jah-SIN-ta | Leahdan | LEE-aun |
| Jarlath | JAR-lath | Lean | LAY-an |
| Junan | JOO-nan | Léan | LAY-an |
| Juanan | JOO-nan | Leanan | LANN-an |
| | | Learai | Larry |
| Kálmán | Kaul-maun | Lelia | LEEL-ya |
| Keara | KEER-a | Líadáin | LEE-a-doyn |
| Kiera | KEER-a | Líadáine | LEE-a-DOYN-yeh |
| Kyran | KEE-ran | Liadaine | LEE-an-yeh |
| | | Liadan | LEE-a-dan |
| Labhrás | Lou-RAUS | Líadán | LEE-dan |
| Labhras | LOUR-as | Liadhnán | LEE-an-aun |
| Lachann | LOK-an | Liam | LEE-am |
| Lachlan | LOK-lan | Life | LIFF-eh |
| Lachlann | LOK-lan | Lil | Lill |

# Pronunciation guide

| | | | |
|---|---|---|---|
| Lila | LEYE-la | Maghnus | MEYE-nus |
| Líle | LEE-la | Mahon | MAH-on |
| Lochlainn | LUK-lin | Maighread | Ma-REY-ad |
| Lochlann | LUK-lan | Maighréad | Ma-REY-ad |
| Loman | LOH-man | Maille | MOLL-yeh |
| Lomán | LOH-maun | Mailse | MOLL-sheh |
| Lonan | LOH-nan | Mailti | MOLL-tee |
| Lonán | Lo-NAUN | Mainchín | MON-keen |
| Lorcan | LUR-kan | Maire | MAH-ree |
| Lorcán | LUR-kaun | Máire | MAU-rah |
| Loretta | Lo-RETT-ah | Mairead | Ma-REYD |
| Loretto | Lo-RETT-oh | Mairéad | Ma-REYD |
| Loughlin | LOK-lin | Maired | Mor-ad |
| Lubhrás | LOO-ras | Mairghréad | Ma-REYD |
| Lucius | LOO-shus | Máirín | MAU-reen |
| Lugh | LOO | Mairin | MAU-reen |
| Lughaidh | LOO-ee | Máirtín | MAUR-teen |
| Lúí | LOO-ee | Maitiú | MOT-yoo |
| Luighseach | LEE-sah | Majella | Ma-JELL-ah |
| Luíseach | LEE-shah | Malachy | MAL-a-kee |
| Lysagh | LEYE-sa | Mallaidh | MOLL-ee |
| | | Malone | Ma-LOHN |
| **M**ac Beatha | Mac-BA-ha | Manchen | MAN-kin |
| Mac Dara | Mac-DARR-eh | Mannix | Manix |
| Macha | MOK-ah | Mánus | MAU-noos |
| Maedóc | MEY-dok | Maodhóg | Ma-HOHG |
| Maeleachlainn | Ma-LOK-lin | Maoilseachlainn | Meel-shok-lan |
| Máelechlainn | Me-LEK-lin | Maolíosa | Ma-LEE-sah |
| Maelisa | Me-LEE-sah | Maolmaodhog | Meyl-MEY-oh |
| Maeve | Meyv | Maolmhuire | Meyl-VIRR-ah |

276

| | | | |
|---|---|---|---|
| Maolra | MEYL-ra | Muirád | Ma-RAUD |
| Maolruaní | Meyl-ROON-ee | Muircheartach | MUR-tah |
| Maraid | Ma-REYD | Muireadhach | MURR-ah |
| Maráid | Ma-RAUD | Muireann | MWIRR-an |
| Mariona | Ma-REE-on-ah | Muirghead | Mirr-EYD |
| Martán | Mar-TAUN | Muirgheal | MIR-gal |
| Mathghamhain | MOH-hoon | Muirinn | MIR-in |
| Mathúin | Moh-OO-in | Muiríoch | Mwir-EE-ok |
| Mave | MEYV | Muiríol | Mwir-EE-ol |
| Meadhbh | MEYV | Muiríos | Mwir-EE-us |
| Meave | MEYV | Muiris | Mwirish |
| Meaveen | MEYV-een | Muirne | MWIR-neh |
| Meibh | MEYV | Munchin | Mun-KEEN |
| Meidhbhín | MEYV-een | Muráid | Ma-RAUD |
| Melaghlin | Meh-LOK-lin | Muraod | Ma-REYD |
| Melissa | Meh-LISS-ah | Murchadh | MUR-ka |
| Meriel | MER-ee-ell | Murel | MYOO-rel |
| Merna | MER-nah | Muriel | MYOO-ree-el |
| Micheál | MEE-haul | Murtagh | MUR-tah |
| Milo | MY-loh | Murtha | MUR-ha |
| Moira | MOY-ra | Myrna | MIR-na |
| Móirín | MOYR-een | | |
| Molais(s)e | Me-LISS-a | Náble | NAUB-lah |
| Mona | MOH-na | Náible | NAUB-leh |
| Monenna | Moh-ENN-ah | Naithí | NAU-hee |
| Mor | More | Naoise | NEE-sheh |
| Mór | More | Naomhán | Ney-VAUN |
| Morainn | MORR-in | Nápla | NAUP-la |
| Morann | MORR-in | Nathí | NAY-thee |
| Muadhnait | MOO-nit | Nathy | NAY-thee |

# Pronunciation guide

| | | | |
|---|---|---|---|
| Naithí | NA-hee | Óengus | EEN-gus |
| Naugher | NOH-er | Ogh(í)e | OH-ee |
| Néamh | Neyv | Oilbhe | OL-veh |
| Neas | Nass | Oilibhéar | Oll-i-vair |
| Neásan | NASS-aun | Oisín | USH-een |
| Neassa | NASS-ah | Oistín | USH-teen |
| Néill | NAY-il | Olave | ULL-av |
| Neill | Neel | Onan | OH-nan |
| Neilla | Neela | Onóra | On-ORE-a |
| Nelda | NELL-da | Oonagh | OO-NA |
| Nia | NEE-ia | Oran | OH-ran |
| Niallán | Neye-LAUN | Órán | OH-ran |
| Niamh | Neev | Órfhlaith | OR-lee |
| Niel | Neel | Orinthia | Or-INTH-ee-ah |
| Nigel | NEYE-jel | Orla | OR-la |
| Noghor | NOH-hor | Orlagh | OR-la |
| Nohor | NOH-hor | Orlaith | OR-lee |
| Nóinín | NOH-neen | Orna | OR-na |
| Nóirín | NOH-reen | Osgar | USS-gar |
| Nolan | NOH-lan | Osheen | USH-een |
| Nollaig | NULL-ig | Ossian | USH-een |
| Nonie | NOH-nee | Ossín | USH-een |
| Nóra | NOH-ra | Ounan | OW-nan |
| Norita | Noh-REE-tah | | |
| Nuala | NOO-ah-lah | **P**adhra | PIE-ra |
| Nyce | NEE-sha | Pádhraic | POY-rik |
| | | Pádhraig | POY-rig |
| **O**dharnait | OHR-nit | Pádraic | PAUD-rik |
| Odhrán | OH-raun | Pádraig | PAUD-rig |
| Odrán | OH-ran | Pádraigín | PAUD-rig-een |

| | | | |
|---|---|---|---|
| Páid | PAU-id | Pierce | PEER-s |
| Páidi | Paddy | Pilib | PI-lib |
| Páidín | PAU-deen | Pól | POHL |
| Paili | PAY-lee | Preanndaigh | PRAN-dee |
| Paití | PAT-ee | Proinséas | PRUN-shee-ass |
| Páraic | PAU-rik | Proinsias | PRUN-shee-as |
| Parthalan | PAR-hal-an | | |
| Parthalán | PAR-hal-aun | Queran | KEER-an |
| Parthalón | PAR-hal-ohn | Quinlevan | QUIN-le-van |
| Párthlán | PAUR-hal-aun | | |
| Pártlán | PAURT-lan | Raghnaid | RYE-nid |
| Partlón | PART-lohn | Raghnailt | RYE-nilt |
| Partnán | PART-naun | Raghnall | RYE-nal |
| Patricia | Pa-TRISH-a | Raidhrí | RYE-ree |
| Peadair | PADH-ar | Ranait | RAH-nit |
| Peadar | PADH-ar | Rannulbh | RAN-ulf |
| Pearce | PEERss | Raonull | RAY-nul |
| Pegeen | Peg-een | Rathnait | RAH-nit |
| Peig | Peg | Reagan | REE-gan, |
| Peigí | Peg-ee | | RAY-gan |
| Peigín | Peg-een | Réamann | RAY-mon |
| Perce | Peer-ss | Reamon | RAY-mon |
| Perse | PEER-ss | Rearden | REER-den |
| Phadrig | FAU-rig | Regan | REE-gan |
| Phaedrig | FAID-rig | Regina | Re-JEEN-ah |
| Phelan | FEE-lan | Reidhrí | RYE-ree |
| Phelim | FEY-lim | Reilly | RYE-lee |
| Phelimy | FEY-lim-ee | Renagh | REE-nah |
| Philomena | Phil-oh-MEE-na | Ríain | REE-an |
| Piaras | PEE-ras | Rian | REE-an |

| | | | |
|---|---|---|---|
| Ribeard | RYE-beard | Rosaleen | ROH-sa-leen |
| Ribeart | RYE-bart | Rosalie | ROH-sa-lee |
| Ribirt | RYE-birt | Rosanna(h) | Roh-san-ah |
| Riobárt | REE-baurt | Roseanna(h) | Roh-san-ah |
| Riobart | REE-bart | Rosheen | ROH-sheen |
| Riocard | RIK-art | Rosina | Roh-ZEEN-ah |
| Rioghnach | REE-nah | Rowan | Roh-an |
| Ríona | REE-nah | Ruadan | ROO-dan |
| Riona | REE-oh-na | Ruadhan | ROO-an |
| Ríonach | REE-nah | Ruaidhrí | ROO-ree |
| Ríordáin | REER-doyn | Ruairí | ROO-ree |
| Risderd | RISH-derd | Ruan | ROO-an |
| Ristéard | RISH-TAIRD | Rúanhnait | ROO-nit |
| Rodan | RO-dan | | |
| Roden | RO-den | **S**adhbh | SIVE (to |
| Rodhlaidhe | ROH-lee | | rhyme with |
| Rodhlann | ROH-laan | | 'alive') |
| Roibeard | RIB-ard | Saidhbhín | SEYE-veen |
| Roibeárd | RIB-aurd | Samhairle | SOR-lee |
| Roibín | Rob-EEN | Saoirse | SEER-she |
| Róis | Roh-ish | Saraid | SOR-id |
| Roisin | Roh-sheen | Sárán | SAUR-aun |
| Róisín | Roh-sheen | Sárnait | SAUR-nit |
| Rónait | ROH-nit | Séafra | SHAY-fra |
| Ronan | ROH-nan | Séafraid | SHAY-frid |
| Rónán | ROH-naun | Séafraidh | SHAY-free |
| Ronit | ROH-nit | Seaghán | SHAUN |
| Rónnad | ROH-nad | Séamas | SHAY-mas |
| Rory | ROH-ree | Séamuisín | SHAY-mush-EEN |
| Rosa | ROH-za | Seamus | SHAY-mus |

| | | | |
|---|---|---|---|
| Séamus | SHAY-mus | Shannagh | SHAN-ah |
| Sean | SHAUN | Shaughan | SHAUN |
| Seán | SHAUN | Shavawn | Sha-VAUN |
| Seanach | SHAN-ok | Shavon(n) | Sha-VON |
| Seanán | Shah-NAUN | Shavonne | Sha-VON |
| Seanchán | Shan-KAUN | Shea | SHAY |
| Seantaigh | SHAN-tee | Sheary | SHEE-ree |
| Séarlait | SHAIR-lat | Sheela(h) | SHEE-la |
| Séarlas | SHAIR-las | Sheelagh | SHEE-la |
| Séarlus | SHAIR-lus | Sheila(h) | SHEE-la |
| Séartha | SHAIR-ha | Sheile | SHEE-leh |
| Séarthra | SHAIR-rah | Shela | SHEE-lah |
| Searthún | SHA-roon | Shelagh | SHEE-lah |
| Seathrún | SHA-roon | Shelegh | SHEE-leh |
| Séathrún | SHAY-roon | Shena | SHEE-nah |
| Séimí | SHAY-mee | Shevaun | Sheh-VON |
| Selia | SEEL-ya | Shevon | Sheh-VON |
| Senan | SENN-an | Shivaun | Shi-VAUN |
| Seoirse | SHORE-she | Shivon(ne) | Shi-VON |
| Seón | SHONE | Shovon | Sho-VON |
| Seorsa | SHORE-sa | Sibby | SIB-ee |
| Seosaimhín | SHOH-sa-feen | Sibéal | Sib-AIL |
| Seosamh | SHOH-saf | Síle | SHEE-leh |
| Seosap(h) | SHOH-saf | Simidh | SHIH-mee |
| Seumas | SHOO-muss | Sinan | SEYE-nan |
| Seumus | SHOO-muss | Síne | SHEEN-ah |
| Shaela | SHAY-la | Sine | SHIN-ah |
| Shahla | SHAH-la | Sinead | Shin-AID |
| Shaila | SHAY-la | Sinéad | Shin-AID |
| Shanna(h) | SHAN-ah | Sineaid | SHIN-AID |

# Pronunciation guide

| | | | |
|---|---|---|---|
| Sinéidín | Shin-AID-een | Tadhgán | THY-gaun |
| Sinon | SEYE-non | Taidhgín | THY-gheen |
| Siobháinín | Shih-VAUN-een | Taig | THYg |
| Siobhan | Shi-VAUN | Tárlach | THOR-lok |
| Siobhán | Shi-VAUN | Tárnaigh | THOR-nee |
| Síoda | SHEE-da | Teabóid | Ta-BOYD |
| Siofraidh | Shee-free | Teague | Taig |
| Siomaidh | SHUM-EE | Teamhair | Tower |
| Síomaigh | SHEE-mee | Teárlach | TAR-lok |
| Siomataigh | SHUM-a-tee | Teigue | TYEg |
| Sionán | SHUN-aun | Thady | They-dee |
| Siothrún | SHUH-roon | Thuathlaith | HOO-lee |
| Sirideán | SHIR-i-daun | Tiarnach | TEER-nok |
| Siubhán | Shih-VAUN | Tiarnán | TEER-naun |
| Siúi | SHOO-ee | Tiernan | TEER-nan |
| Siún | SHOON | Tighe | TEE |
| Sive | SIVE (rhymes with 'alive') | Tighearnach | TEER-nok |
| | | Tighearnán | TEER-naun |
| Sivney | SIV-nee | Tiobóid | Ti-BOYD |
| Sláine | SLOYN-ye | Toirdhealbhach | TOR-lek |
| Slania | SLON-ya | Toiréasa | Teh-RAY-sah |
| Slanie | SLON-yeh | Tomáisín | Tuh-MAUSH-een |
| Somerled | So-ar-lee | Tomás | Tuh-MAUS |
| Somhairle | SOR-lee | Traoine | TREE-na |
| Sorcha | SOR-ra | Traolach | TREY-luk |
| Sósaidh | SO-see | Treasa | TRAH-sah |
| Suibhne | SIV-neh | Treise | TRESH-eh |
| Synan | SEYE-nan | Trina | TREEN-a |
| | | Triona | TREEN-a |
| Tadgh | TYEg, THYg | Tríona | TREEN-a |

| | | | |
|---|---|---|---|
| Tuathal | Too-hal | Uinseann | IN-sun |
| Tuathla | Too-lah | Ulicia | Uh-LISH-ah |
| Tuilelaith | Too-lee | Ulick | YOO-lik |
| Turlough | TUR-lok | Ultan | UL-tan |
| Tyrone | Tih-RONE | Ulysses | Yoo-liss-aze |
| | | Una | OO-na |
| **U**aine | OO-neh | Úna | OO-na |
| Uainthne | Oo-ee-neh | | |
| Uaitne | Oo-ee-neh | **V**igean | |
| Uilleac | ILL-ak | | |
| Uilleag | ILL-ag | **Y**seult | EE-sult |
| Uilliam | William | | |

# Top 100 Boys' Names 2002

| | | | | | | |
|---|---|---|---|---|---|---|
| 1 | Jack | | | 25 | Oisin | −2 |
| 2 | Sean | | | 26 | Liam | −2 |
| 3 | Adam | | | 27 | Nathan | +5 |
| 4 | Conor | | | 28 | Ciaran | −3 |
| 5 | James | | | 29 | Evan | +1 |
| 6 | Daniel | +5 | | 30 = | Jake | +4 |
| 7 | Cian | −1 | | 30 = | Robert | +3 |
| 8 | Michael | +2 | | 32 | Kevin | +4 |
| 9 | David | −2 | | 33 = | Joseph | +2 |
| 10 | Luke | −1 | | 33 = | Stephen | -7 |
| 11 | Dylan | −3 | | 35 | Alex | +10 |
| 12 | Aaron | | | 36 | Kyle | +17 |
| 13 | Patrick | +4 | | 37 | Jason | +8 |
| 14 | Ryan | +4 | | 38 = | Brian | +1 |
| 15 | John | | | 38 = | Cathal | |
| 16 | Eoin | +2 | | 40 | Niall | +1 |
| 17 | Matthew | +5 | | 41 | Andrew | −4 |
| 18 | Thomas | +4 | | 42 | Jordan | −13 |
| 19 = | Ben | +8 | | 43 | Samuel | +6 |
| 19 = | Joshua | +9 | | 44 | Dean | −9 |
| 21 | Shane | −7 | | 45 | Paul | −2 |
| 22 | Mark | −6 | | 46 | Lee | +1 |
| 23 | Jamie | −3 | | 47 | Christopher | −5 |
| 24 | Darragh | −3 | | 48 | Eoghan | −4 |

| 49 | William | +3 | 74 = | Ross | −11 |
|---|---|---|---|---|---|
| 50 = | Ethan | +1 | 76 | Colm | −5 |
| 50 = | Peter | −2 | 77 | Diarmuid | +6 |
| 52 | Cormac | +7 | 78 | Ian | +9 |
| 53 | Benjamin | +13 | 79 | Keith | −5 |
| 54 | Ronan | −4 | 80 | Tadhg | +8 |
| 55 | Gavin | −1 | 81 | Leon | −13 |
| 56 | Alexander | +9 | 82 = | Jonathan | +4 |
| 57 | Rory | +4 | 82 = | Richard | −7 |
| 58 | Scott | +8 | 84 = | Brendan | +6 |
| 59 | Craig | −19 | 84 = | Owen | −1 |
| 60 = | Alan | −1 | 84 = | Padraig | −5 |
| 60 = | Callum | +16 | 87 | Gary | +11 |
| 62 = | Aidan | +11 | 88 | Finn | +7 |
| 62 = | Josh | +19 | 89 | Edward | −12 |
| 64 | Anthony | −8 | 90 = | Connor | +11 |
| 65 | Killian | −10 | 90 = | Tom | +4 |
| 66 = | Cillian | −8 | 92 | Eric | +14 |
| 66 = | Fionn | +4 | 93 | Charlie | +21 |
| 68 | Harry | −12 | 94 | Oran | +2 |
| 69 | Kieran | +3 | 95 = | Daragh | −15 |
| 70 | Brandon | +13 | 95 = | Denis | +22 |
| 71 | Sam | +18 | 97 = | Dara | −7 |
| 72 | Darren | −10 | 97 = | Lorcan | −4 |
| 73 | Kian | −10 | 99 = | Seamus | +12 |
| 74 = | Martin | −4 | 100 | Steven | +32 |

# Top 100 Girls' Names 2002

| | | | | | | |
|---|---|---|---|---|---|---|
| 1 | Sarah | | | 24 = | Roisin | +1 |
| 2 | Aoife | | | 26 | Ava | +15 |
| 3 | Ciara | +2 | | 27 | Aisling | −4 |
| 4 | Emma | −1 | | 28 | Ella | +20 |
| 5 | Chloe | −1 | | 29 | Grace | −2 |
| 6 | Amy | +2 | | 30 | Sinead | +3 |
| 7 | Katie | +2 | | 31 | Saoirse | −3 |
| 8 | Niamh | −2 | | 32 | Tara | |
| 9 | Sophie | +7 | | 33 | Molly | −2 |
| 10 | Lauren | −4 | | 34 | Jennifer | +5 |
| 11 | Megan | −1 | | 35 | Holly | +14 |
| 12 | Hannah | +3 | | 36 | Lucy | −1 |
| 13 | Rachel | −2 | | 37 | Shannon | −8 |
| 14 | Rebecca | | | 38 | Caitlin | −4 |
| 15 | Leah | −3 | | 39 | Aine | −3 |
| 16 | Laura | −3 | | 40 | Orla | −2 |
| 17 | Jessica | +3 | | 41 | Mary | −4 |
| 18 | Kate | +4 | | 42 | Jade | −12 |
| 19 | Emily | −1 | | 43 = | Eimear | −3 |
| 20 | Caoimhe | −1 | | 43 = | Zoe | −1 |
| 21 | Anna | +5 | | 45 | Clodagh | −3 |
| 22 | Shauna | −5 | | 46 | Ellie | +43 |
| 23 | Ellen | +1 | | 47 | Mia | +25 |
| 24 = | Nicole | −3 | | 48 = | Erin | −1 |

| | | | | | |
|---|---|---|---|---|---|
| 48 = | Louise | +2 | 75 | Maeve | −5 |
| 50 | Eva | −6 | 76 | Alice | +11 |
| 51 | Abbie | +13 | 77 | Isabelle | +27 |
| 52 | Katelyn | | 78 = | Alexandra | −10 |
| 53 | Maria | +5 | 78 = | Jane | |
| 54 | Claire | −10 | 80 = | Alanna | −6 |
| 55 = | Alannah | −3 | 80 = | Lara | −37 |
| 55 = | Lisa | | 82 | Emer | +2 |
| 57 | Kelly | +12 | 83 = | Courtney | +1 |
| 58 | Catherine | −4 | 83 = | Victoria | −17 |
| 59 | Eve | −12 | 85 = | Andrea | |
| 60 | Alison | +2 | 85 = | Lily | +6 |
| 61 | Michelle | +1 | 87 = | Siobhan | −12 |
| 62 | Elizabeth | −2 | 87 = | Zara | −4 |
| 63 = | Fiona | +11 | 89 = | Nadine | +54 |
| 63 = | Robyn | −12 | 89 = | Rachael | −10 |
| 65 | Abby | −12 | 91 = | Charlotte | −4 |
| 66 = | Aimee | +8 | 91 = | Sara | −7 |
| 66 = | Danielle | −8 | 93 | Heather | +19 |
| 68 = | Abigail | −2 | 94 = | Ailbhe | +13 |
| 68 = | Kayleigh | +6 | 94 = | Isabel | +35 |
| 68 = | Ruth | +12 | 94 = | Michaela | −24 |
| 71 = | Grainne | −5 | 94 = | Sadhbh | +9 |
| 71 = | Olivia | −10 | 94 = | Stephanie | −3 |
| 73 | Jodie | −1 | 99 | Eabha | +61 |
| 74 | Leanne | −18 | 100 | Laoise | +13 |

# Further reading

## Names

*Irish Names* Donnachadh Ó Corráin & Fidelma Maguire (Dublin 1990). The most scholarly book on the subject, it contains fascinating information and is reliable in its treatment of the language but deals only with early names and can be difficult to use.

*Irish Names for Children* Patrick Woulfe (Dublin 1923; out of print). First book of its kind and still useful.

*Irish Christian Names* Ronan Coughlan (London 1979). Takes a refreshingly broad view of what an Irish name is, but has been criticised for inaccuracies.

*The Surnames of Ireland* Edward MacLysaght (Dublin 1985). The standard work on Irish surnames.

*Unusual and Most Popular Baby Names* Cleveland Kent Evans & the American Name Society (Illinois 1994). Useful for information on usage in the USA.

## People and Myth

*Myth, Legend and Romance: An Encyclopaedia of the Irish Folk Tradition* Daithi Ó hÓgáin (London 1990); *A Dictionary of Irish Mythology* Peter Berresford Ellis (Oxford 1991) are both wonderful sources of stories. *The Irish Saints* Daphne D.C. Pochin Mould (Dublin 1964) discusses a number of Irish saints. *The Oxford Dictionary of Saints* David Hugh Farmer (Oxford 1978) covers a wider range more briefly.